HISTOLOGY
AN IDENTIFICATION MANUAL

HISTOLOGY
AN IDENTIFICATION MANUAL

Robert B. Tallitsch, Ph.D.

Augustana College
Rock Island, Illinois

Ronald S. Guastaferri, B.A., M.A.M.S.

Art Coordinator and Illustrator

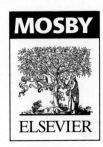

MOSBY

ELSEVIER

MOSBY
ELSEVIER

1600 John F. Kennedy Blvd.
Ste 1800
Philadelphia, PA 19103-2899

HISTOLOGY: AN IDENTIFICATION MANUAL   ISBN: 978-0-323-04955-9

Notice

Knowledge and best practice in this field are constantly changing. As new research and experience broaden our knowledge, changes in practice, treatment and drug therapy may become necessary or appropriate. Readers are advised to check the most current information provided (i) on procedures featured or (ii) by the manufacturer of each product to be administered, to verify the recommended dose or formula, the method and duration of administration, and contraindications. It is the responsibility of the practitioner, relying on their own experience and knowledge of the patient, to make diagnoses, to determine dosages and the best treatment of each individual patient, and to take all appropriate safety precautions. To the fullest extent of the law, neither the Publisher nor the Author assumes any liability for any injury and/or damage to persons or property arising out of or related to any use of the material contained in this book.

The Publisher

Library of Congress Cataloging-in-Publication Data
Tallitsch, Robert B.
   Histology: an identification manual / Robert B. Tallitsch; Ronald S. Guastaferri, art coordinator and illustrator.— 1st ed.
       p. ; cm.
   Includes bibliographical references and index.
   ISBN-13: 978-0-323-04955-9
   1.   Histology—Laboratory manuals.
   [DNLM: 1.   Histological Techniques—Laboratory Manuals.   2.   Tissues—ultrastructure—Laboratory Manuals. QS 525 T149h 2009]   I. Guastaferri, Ronald S.   II. Title.
   QM555.T35 2009
   611'.018078—dc22

                                                    2007023489

Acquisitions Editor: Kate Dimock
Developmental Editor: Christine Abshire
Project Manager: Mary B. Stermel
Design Direction: Charles Gray
Marketing Manager: Alyson Sherby

Printed in China

Last digit is the print number: 9   8   7   6   5   4   3   2   1

Dedication

This text is dedicated to all of the Augustana students
I have had the pleasure of teaching during my time here
at Augustana College and to Mary, Steven, and Molly for
tolerating the long hours needed to accomplish this dream.

Robert B. Tallitsch

To Bob, for bringing me on board,
and to Kris, Sophie, and Bella (who keep me afloat).

Ronald Guastaferri

Preface

The more I taught histology, the more my students and I came to realize that most histology atlases are "picture books" containing illustrations, photomicrographs, and captions explaining what the tissue was and what could be seen. However, regardless of the atlas I used in class, something always seemed to be missing. *No atlas presented a way for students to learn histology—to learn how to identify an unknown histological specimen.* The more my students and I talked, the more I came to realize that someone needed to write a textbook that did just that—taught students how to identify histological specimens. As a result of my students' prodding and suggestions, this text came to be.

This atlas is designed to help students to develop the investigative skills needed to identify an unknown histological preparation. All the details and theories presented in a histology class are useless if students can't correctly identify a specimen. This textbook is not intended to stand alone; rather, it is to be used in conjunction with accompanying lecture resources, as well as with material presented in lecture by the professor. The lecture and handouts will present the cellular biology and ultrastructure that are essential in a histology course.

Therefore, in order to meet our stated goals, this book is organized in the following manner:

- **Content:** This book contains material that is typically taught in a *first* histology course, whether at the undergraduate or graduate/professional school level. In addition, material normally found in comprehensive histology textbooks is not repeated here. Detailed descriptions of function, ultrastructure, or current research findings are therefore not included.

- **Terminology:** Histologists are notorious for not having a uniform and universally accepted terminology. However, in this book we have expended great effort to incorporate the terminology endorsed by the International Federation of Associations of Anatomists as published in the 1998 *Terminologia Anatomica* (T.A.). In addition, we have tried to incorporate as much as possible of the new terminology published in the first edition (2008) of the *Terminologia Histologica: International Terms for Human Cytology and Histology* (TH). However, if we have missed one or more of the new terms, you have our apologies, and we will do our best to correct any omissions in subsequent editions. Because it will take some time for the newly accepted terminology to become universal in its usage, we have, where applicable, provided the older terminology in parentheses.

- **Figure Reference Locators:** The reader will note that figure callouts are in a different color from the rest of the paragraph (Figure 1-1). This design will help you to mark your spot as you move from text to figure and then back to the text.

- **Photomicrographs:** As you progress from the four basic tissues to organ systems, the manner in which you examine histological preparations should change. Oil-immersion and high-dry objectives are used less frequently, and scanning power is used more frequently. Therefore photomicrographs presented early in the text were taken using some combination of low, medium, and high power. However, as you progress through the text, the appearance of photomicrographs taken with high-power or oil-immersion lenses becomes less and less frequent, thereby matching the normal progression of specimen examination in a typical histology class.

- **Artifacts and Staining:** The photomicrographs in this textbook are presented in a format that will be close to what you will encounter in the laboratory. Most specimens were taken from standard student sets, so there will be very few photomicrographs with exotic stains that would seldom, if ever, be seen in the laboratory. In addition, specimens with artifacts, variations attributable to plane of section, specimen thickness, and staining imperfections are included. *We hope that the photomicrographs included in this text will therefore approximate what you will actually see in the laboratory more than any other atlas available at this time.*

- **Pen-and-Ink Drawings:** First-time histology students often have a difficult time focusing their attention on the most important details of a specimen. As Ron Guastaferri and I pieced together this book, we spent a considerable amount of time discussing what students need to know to be able to correctly identify each specimen presented. We decided which details should and should not be included in each of Ron's line drawings that accompany the photomicrographs in this text. *As a result, not every detail is repeated in the pen-and-ink drawings—only those that are essential for the learning and identification process.* The field of view of a particular drawing will replicate exactly what is shown in the corresponding photomicrograph, even though not all elements of the photo will be represented with the same amount of detail in the drawing. The student should use these pen-and-ink drawings as "road maps" to navigate the photomicrographs. They should help students develop the ability to quickly scan and identify key structures on any specimen slide.

- **Labels:** All too often, the placement of labels on photomicrographs or illustrations obscures important structures. Therefore all photomicrographs are unlabelled. Labels, where needed, are found on the accompanying pen-and-ink illustration. Anything labeled on the pen-and-ink illustration will be found in *italics* within the description of the photomicrograph.

- **Lack of Label Repetition:** As a teacher and an author I assume that students will remember what was covered earlier in my course or in the textbook. Granted, repetition is important for learning—but so is self-testing. Therefore material that has been covered in chapters dealing with the four basic tissues is not labeled later in the text. For instance, the histological characteristics of smooth muscle are covered in Chapter 6. Therefore when smooth muscle is encountered in a subsequent chapter (such as Chapter 16, Gastrointestinal System) it is not labeled on the pen-and-ink drawings. However, the first time the student encounters a reference to smooth muscle in Chapter 16, the student is referred back to the appropriate section within Chapter 6 for review of the histological characteristics of smooth muscle. Students at Augustana who have used in-class versions of this material have found this teaching pedagogy to be quite effective for the retention of important material. Indeed, it was my histology students who convinced me to eliminate labels for material covered in the chapters dealing with the four basic tissues that is repeated later in the text.

- **Text:** I have done my best to make the text student friendly. Therefore important items are presented in bulleted lists throughout the book as much as possible. In addition, important identification features of the tissues and organs discussed are listed in *italics* for easy and quick reference.

- **Commonly Misidentified Tissues:** Since my first histology class at Augustana, I have been accumulating a list of mistakes made by students on laboratory examinations. As a result of this list, I have been able to compile a series of boxes entitled "Commonly Misidentified Tissues" within various chapters of this book. These boxes review the histological characteristics of tissues that are similar in appearance and that therefore may be easily misidentified. These tips are intended to help prevent students from repeating these common mistakes.

- **Study Tips:** Students are presented with a series of suggestions that will aid them in developing a solid studying methodology.

- **Logic Trees:** Students are given a logical series of steps that will help them to arrive at a correct identification of an unknown specimen. These steps are organized into a series of simple "yes" or "no" questions that should help the student to pursue a line of logical thinking that will aid in the identification of an unknown specimen.

Finally, this textbook is not the product of only one person's labor. Special thanks must be given to a wide range of individuals, without whom this book never would have come to fruition.

- Anne Madura Earel—my very first "editor" for this text while she was a student at Augustana. Anne helped by editing the first rough draft that was pieced together more than 7 years ago.

- Kathryn Gray—another student editor from Augustana. Kat's input was timely and extremely valuable as this project neared completion.

- Ron Guastaferri—friend, former student, and illustrator beyond compare! Ron saw and understood my vision for this book from the first, and jumped in with no questions asked. Ron—you stuck with me through thick and thin and held on to the vision of this project when others would have jumped ship. Without your excellent artistic work, input, and patience, this book never could have made the transition from idea to reality.

- All the histology students whom I have had the pleasure of teaching at Augustana since I joined the faculty in 1975. Without their initial suggestions and prodding, I never would have put together the first manual, nor would I have created a prospectus. Even though it has been a while, I would like to give special thanks to those first students who suggested I write a histology atlas way back in the spring semester of 1984.

    Bill Hoover, M.D. (class of '84)

    Krista Dutton Scoggins, D.V.M. (class of '85)

    Sonya Eiben Mariano, M.D. (class of '85)

    Pete Vienne, M.D. (class of '85)

- The various students from my histology classes throughout the years who have performed "field tests" on various aspects of this text as it was being formulated in my mind—especially the histology classes of the spring semesters of the 2002–2003 and 2005–2006 academic years. Your input was valuable and resulted in numerous additions and alterations in the final project. Thank you!

As you read through this book, please be sure to contact me with any and all corrections, questions, and suggestions.

    Bob Tallitsch

    Professor of Biology

    Augustana College

    Rock Island, IL 61201-2296

    RobertTallitsch@augustana.edu

Contents

Chapter **1**

GETTING STARTED

Chapter Objectives

This chapter is designed to help you do exactly what the title says—get started. Therefore it is intended to:

1. Present some generic information on the use of a brightfield microscope. Your instructor will provide additional information, but this brief introduction should enable you to get started with minimal difficulty.

2. Point out techniques that may be used to maximize the information retained as you view histological specimens in the laboratory.

3. Provide tips that will facilitate the process of identifying an unknown histological specimen.

To the new student of histology, the process of identifying an unknown histological specimen may seem daunting. Current texts and atlases are filled with endless details of microscopic anatomy as seen with light microscopes and electron microscopes. In addition, most atlases simply present pictures of histological specimens with labels indicating the source of the specimen, magnification, stains used, and various items of interest on the photomicrograph. *Yet the questions of a beginning histology student have not been answered—namely, "What is the specimen and how do I figure that out?"* Few, if any, tips are provided that will aid in learning how to identify an unknown histological specimen. This process is typically left for students to discern on their own; hence my incentive to write this book. *Students of histology need a laboratory book that instructs them in the process of identifying an unknown histological specimen.* This book was not written as a typical histology atlas. *Rather, this book was written to help teach you how to interpret and identify unknown histological specimens.* Therefore the photomicrographs in this book are presented in a format that will be very close to that which you will encounter in the laboratory. Specimens with artifacts, variations attributable to the plane of section, specimen thickness, and staining imperfections are included. *Therefore we hope that the photomicrographs included in this book will approximate what you will actually see in the laboratory.*

Use of a Brightfield Microscope

The following material is generic, that is, it is not written for any particular brand or style of light microscope. Even if you are familiar with the use of a microscope, you should read the following material.

Microscope Placement and Utilization

Use both hands when carrying a microscope. One hand should have a firm grip on the arm of the microscope, and the other should support the microscope from underneath. *Never, under any circumstances, carry a microscope with one hand or carry two microscopes at one time.*

Provide ample space before placing the microscope on the desk. *Never, under any circumstances, slide the microscope across the laboratory bench.* If you need to change the position of the microscope, pick up the instrument and place it in the new location. The vibrations caused by sliding the microscope across the laboratory bench may have an adverse effect on the microscope's optics.

If the microscope has inclined eyepieces and a rotating head, you have two options for positioning the instrument. However you choose to use the instrument, the head should be rotated so that the eyepieces are pointing toward the arm of the microscope when the instrument is being carried or placed back in storage.

Lens Care

It is important that the light, condenser, and objective lenses be kept clean to allow the maximal amount of light to enter the microscope. The light, condenser, and objective lenses should be cleaned only with high-quality lens paper or cotton swabs and a high-quality glass-cleaning solution.

Objectives

Change objectives by rotating the revolving nosepiece on the microscope. *To prevent damage to the objective's threads, never change magnification by grasping the objective!* All objectives on the microscope are to be cleaned only with a high-quality glass-cleaning solution and either high-quality lens paper or clean cotton swabs.

Eyepieces

To test the eyepiece for cleanliness, rotate it between your thumb and forefinger as you look at a well-focused slide through the microscope. A rotating pattern will be evidence of dirt on the eyepiece. Eye makeup and natural oils from eyelashes will contribute to dirt on microscope eyepieces. Clean the eyepiece first with a cotton swab that has been lightly dampened with a high-quality glass-cleaning solution. Then dry the eyepiece, either with a dry cotton swab or dry, high-quality lens paper.

Condenser and Diaphragm

The condenser should be at its highest point without touching the slide. If a pattern shows in the visual field, lower the condenser (or clean it) until the pattern disappears.

Under most circumstances, the diaphragm should be kept approximately halfway open. The amount of light desired should be regulated by altering the brightness of the light source rather than by altering the setting of the diaphragm. The diaphragm setting should be changed only to increase the contrast and depth of field of the specimen.

Initial Specimen Examination

Before placing a specimen on the microscope stage, examine the slide with the naked eye by holding it up to the light. This will allow you to do two things before examining the specimen under the microscope: (1) determine the cleanliness of the slide, and (2) determine the general orientation of the specimen.

Focusing and Low-Power Examination

The low-power objective of the microscope is used to gain a general orientation to a new slide. *It should be the first objective used to view every preparation.*

To focus the microscope, it is necessary to alter the distance between the slide and the objective lens. You accomplish this with knobs on the side of the microscope. On some instruments, these knobs cause the objective lens to move up and down in relation to the stage. On other microscopes, the objective lens is stationary and the stage is moved. In either case, the larger knob is used when coarse focusing is desired. The smaller knob is used for fine focusing.

When focusing, consideration must be given to the *working distance* of the lens. This is the distance between the lens and the slide when the specimen is in sharp focus. The greater the power of an objective, the smaller its working distance. Note that an oil-immersion lens may have a working distance of only 0.14 mm. This amounts to a 0.005-inch clearance between the lens and slide! If a slide with a thick cover glass is used, the actual working distance will be even less; therefore you must exercise care when using high-dry and oil-immersion lenses. (See the Oil-Immersion Techniques section.) *Although most microscopes have built-in mechanisms to prevent damage to the oil-immersion lens, the safest procedure is to make it a rule never to use the coarse focus adjustment while looking into the microscope if you are using anything other than the lowest-power objective.*

When examining a specimen, *always* start with the low-power (usually 10×) objective. Mount the slide in the mechanical stage slide holder with the cover glass up. While looking through the eyepieces, rotate the coarse focus until the specimen begins to come into focus. Then, *while using only the fine focus knob*, slowly bring the specimen completely into focus. As you rotate to other objectives to view the specimen, *only the fine focus knob will be needed. Never use the coarse focusing knob with any objective other than low power!*

High-Dry Examination

Once the microscopic field has been surveyed to locate the specimen and an overall orientation of the specimen has been obtained, you can change the magnification to an intermediate power or to high dry, depending on the size of the field to be studied. If the specimen is in focus with low power (10×), all that is necessary to change lenses is to rotate the nosepiece so that the desired lens is locked into place. Because most microscopes are parfocal, it can be assumed that the specimen under the new lens will be either in focus or nearly so. *You must remember that once you have switched from the lower-power objective, you should adjust the focus only with the fine focus knob!*

Oil-Immersion Techniques

For certain slides and preparations you will need to use the oil-immersion lens. However, once you become more comfortable looking at tissue sections, you will use this objective less and less. In this book we will point out those sections that should be viewed under oil immersion; therefore it is not necessary to use oil immersion unless it is suggested.

The greatest difficulty students have with this lens is that its working distance is so small that incorrect focusing techniques will result in broken cover glasses or slides. These objectives are the most expensive ones on the microscope, so it is essential that you observe certain safeguards.

One of the easiest and safest ways to use the oil-immersion objective is to progress from low power to medium power and then to oil immersion. This is accomplished by bypassing the high-dry objective. After a good viewing section of the slide is obtained, rotate the fine focus knob so that the stage (or lens, depending on the design of the microscope) is moved *away from the slide.* (It is best to perform this step with the scanning lens in place to prevent damage to the slide should you rotate the coarse-adjustment knob in the wrong direction.) After moving the objective a safe distance from the stage, place a small drop of immersion oil on the slide in the center of the current field of vision and swing the oil-immersion objective into place. Carefully raise the stage (or lower the objective) *while watching the slide from the side.* Continue until the objective *just touches the oil droplet.* Now look through the eyepiece and bring the specimen into focus using the *fine adjustment only.* Adjust the light intensity if necessary.

When another slide is to be examined, start moving the oil objective out of the immersion oil with the fine focus *while watching the slide from the side.* When the lens is out of the oil, continue to move the objective away from the slide with the coarse adjustment while also continuing to watch the slide from the side. *Always* clean the slide carefully before returning it to its storage location. In addition, always clean the oil-immersion objective *after every use;* never allow oil to remain on the lens. Clean the objective and slide by first removing any excess oil with a clean, dry cotton swab. Then clean the lens and slide using a cotton swab moistened with a high-quality glass cleaner. Finally, dry the lens and slide with a new, clean, dry cotton swab.

Additional Suggestions

Check the bottle of immersion oil to make certain it is not cloudy. The oil should be completely clear.

You must be careful never to lower the high-dry objective into the immersion oil. Doing so would damage the seal around the lens and cause oil to leak into the housing, permanently damaging the lens.

How to Interpret Tissue Sections

Correlate Structure and Function

Histology is defined by *Stedman's Medical Dictionary*[1] as "the science concerned with the minute structure of cells, tissues, and organs in relation to their function." However, from a practical point of view, histology is more than just the structure of cells, tissues, and organs. It also involves the identification of unknown specimens—*the process of learning how to determine what it is you are looking at and why.* This section provides several suggestions that will allow you to start developing a logical process of identifying an unknown histological preparation.

It is important to keep in mind that the interpretation of histological sections cannot occur in isolation. *When* you take a course in histology is unimportant. Whether or not histology is part of an entry-level course in the biological sciences, taken as a senior-level college course, or taken as part of the curriculum of a first-year medical student, it is essential that histology students try to correlate what they have learned or are learning in anatomy, physiology, and other courses and use that information as

they work to correctly identify an unknown specimen. As a student of histology you must:

- Remember the three-dimensional anatomical characteristics of the organ that was the source for the histological section. How might the shape of the organ affect its histological appearance when sectioned? What other organs, blood vessels, and ducts are normally found in close proximity to the organ being sectioned? How might these structures aid you in identifying the tissue section currently on your microscope stage?

- Learn to relate structure and function. The ultrastructure of any tissue or organ is tightly coupled to its function. Even if you have yet to take a physiology course, it is important to try to relate the physiological functions of every tissue, organ, and organ system to its histological structure. Trying to understand histological structure in isolation will increase the likelihood of confusion and frustration. However, studying the histological structure of a tissue or organ in conjunction with its physiological function will lead to logical conclusions and relationships that will make specimen identification considerably easier.

- As you make the transition from the four basic tissues to organs and then to organ systems, remember the ultrastructure of the "typical" cells of that organ (secretory cells, transport cells, and so forth). In addition, remember specific cellular structures that are enhanced by the particular stains used in the preparation of the tissue in question (see Appendix). Finally, tying these and other pieces of information together provides you with valuable insights into the histological appearances of many structures that you will be identifying throughout your histology course.

Tissue Preparation, Histochemistry, and Cytochemistry

In order to correlate structure and function it is important to have at least a rudimentary understanding of the process used in the preparation of histological specimens.

Tissue Preparation

Tissues that were photographed for this book were obtained from standard student histology slide sets. Most of these tissues were fixed in formalin, embedded in paraffin, and then stained with hematoxylin and eosin (H & E).

Fixation is a process in which cell metabolism is stopped and tissue structure is preserved. The most commonly used preservative is formalin (37% solution of formaldehyde) in combination with a variety of buffers.

In order to slice specimens thinly enough (5 to 15 μm) to allow the transmission of light through the specimen, the tissue must first be *embedded* in a suitable medium. Such embedding facilitates the straight, thin cutting of the specimen. Preserved tissues that are to be embedded must first be washed and then soaked in progressively stronger alcohol solutions until the specimen finally is soaked in a solution of 100% alcohol. This process allows the tissue to dehydrate (that is, water has been removed) and also removes all intracellular and extracellular alcohol-soluble compounds, including fat, glycogen, proteoglycans, ions, intermediary metabolites, glucose, and mucous. Following dehydration with alcohol, the tissue is soaked in an organic solvent (typically toluene or xylol) to remove all of the alcohol from the specimen. This process also facilitates the penetration of the embedding medium (typically hot paraffin) deep into the tissue specimen. After the paraffin has cooled, the block of paraffin is sectioned, and the resulting thin slices are mounted on a microscope slide.

Staining is the final step in the preparation of tissue samples. Before staining, the specimen is again soaked in an organic solvent to remove all of the paraffin from the tissue. The specimen is then rehydrated by progressive soaking in solutions that simultaneously contain less and less alcohol and more and more water.

Chemical Composition of Tissue Samples Ready for Staining

As a result of the fixation process, the tissue that has been mounted on the microscope slide has a chemical composition significantly different from that found within living tissues. The chemicals remaining in biological tissues after fixation are mainly large macromolecules that are not alcohol soluble, such as membrane phospholipid-protein compounds, membrane phospholipid-carbohydrate compounds, extracellular proteins, intracellular cytoskeleton proteins, and nucleoproteins.

Chemical Basis of Staining

H & E is the most commonly used stain in histology. Eosin is an acidic dye and therefore has a net negative charge. Similarly, hematoxylin, a basic dye, carries a net positive charge. Acidic dyes interact with the cationic groups found intracellularly and extracellularly, while basic dyes interact with the anionic groups. A partial listing of those tissue components that interact with acidic and basic dyes is given below:

- Basophilic tissue components (components that interact with basic dyes such as hematoxylin) include the following:

  - Extracellular carbohydrates, such as those found in cartilage

  - Nucleic acids within the nucleus and nucleolus

  - Cytoplasmic components of the rough endoplasmic reticulum

- Acidophilic tissue components (components that interact with acidic dyes such as eosin) include the following:

  - Cytoplasmic filaments

  - Intracellular membrane components

  - Extracellular fibers

Maximize Your Field of Vision

Beginning students of histology tend to spend too much time using the high-dry or oil objectives. This is a natural inclination; the beginning histology student assumes that the higher magnification power will reveal more information about a specimen.

Although this inclination may prove to be correct in some instances, it is often the case that more valuable information will be obtained by examining a specimen with the low- or medium-power objectives than with the high-power or oil-immersion objectives. Note how the field of vision decreases significantly as the magnification of the following photomicrographs increases from 25× to 50× to 100× (**Figures 1-1 to 1-3**). A histological identification is made by taking into account *all* of the characteristics of each portion of the specimen being viewed—understanding the "big picture" of the specimen in question. You will see these all-inclusive characteristics only by using the lower-power objectives. Remember—the higher the magnification power of the objective, the smaller the field of vision. It is difficult to make a correct identification by spending the majority of your time using high-power objectives.

In addition to maximizing use of the low-power objectives when identifying an unknown specimen, keep the following suggestions in mind:

- Do not depend totally on specimen colors. Yes, staining characteristics are important, but you must learn how to rely on the structural characteristics of the tissue in addition to its staining characteristics.

- Try to develop a mental picture of the specimen being studied. This can be facilitated by drawing pictures of the specimens studied in the laboratory.

- Study unknown specimens in a manner that enables you to list a minimum of three reasons for your identification of the specimen. These reasons should be the type that can be documented in a standard histology text.

The identification of an unknown slide is similar to a mystery story. You are given a series of clues that you must understand, analyze, and use in order to make a correct identification. Memorization will not work! You need to develop some methodology that will enable you to logically progress through the various options and arrive at the correct answer. Throughout this book, we plan to provide these logical choices for you—in both verbal and picture format. As you progress through your first histology course, you may choose to use the methodology outlined in this book or you may develop some alternative form of your own. The approach used in this book is one in which you force yourself to think in a series of simple "yes" and "no" questions. To help you to start thinking in this manner, we have included numerous "Logic Trees" throughout the book. Look these over and use them if they help you in your identification process. If you feel more comfortable with another methodology, good! The important things are that you have (or develop) a methodology that works and that you then consistently use this methodology to properly identify an unknown specimen.

Interpreting Planes of Section

Two of the most frustrating things a beginning histology student encounters are lumped under the general category of "artifact"—something that you may see on a specimen that is not a normal component of that tissue or organ. Fixation, staining, and mounting techniques may produce artifacts in the specimen. Some artifacts may aid in the identification of a specimen, while others may

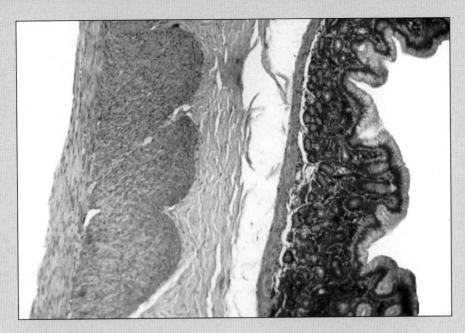

Figure 1-1 (25×): Fundic stomach.

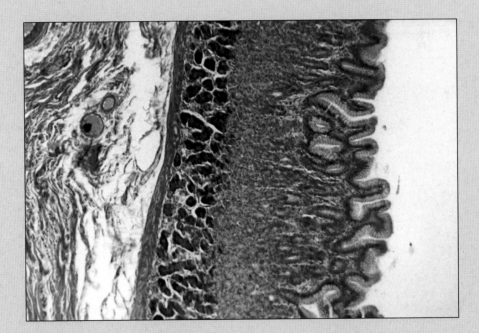

Figure 1-2 (50×): Fundic stomach.

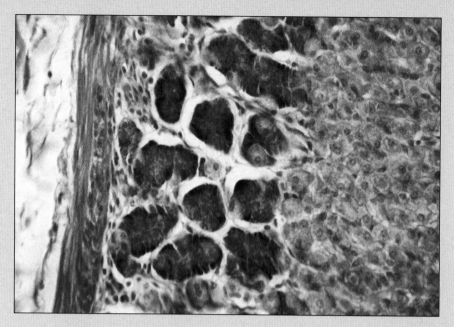

Figure 1-3 (100×): Fundic stomach.

hinder it. Only experience will enable you to learn how to ignore some artifacts and pay attention to others. In addition, the plane of section will vary from specimen to specimen, as well as from structure to structure within a specimen, thereby giving rise to "sectioning artifacts." As you look at a slide, it is important to pay attention to the plane of section. Is the preparation being examined a cross, longitudinal, or oblique section? As you look at Figures 1-4 to 1-7, note how varying planes of section will alter the view of the structures in question. The appearance of a femur (Figure 1-4), curved tube (Figure 1-5), and lemon (Figure 1-6)

will vary depending on the plane of section. Similarly, the structures that are visible will vary depending on the level of sectioning. Figure 1-7 demonstrates how the plane of section will alter the view of a tissue depending on the level of the sectioning. There is no quick way to learn which artifacts are important to remember and which are important to ignore. To aid you in this learning process, we have deliberately incorporated micrographs in this book that contain sectioning and staining artifacts. When present, they are discussed in the body of the text.

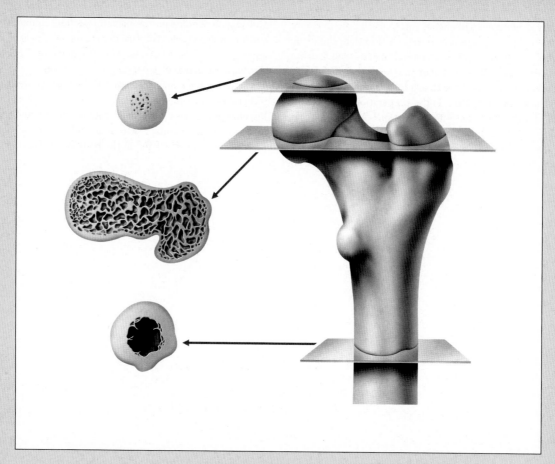

Figure 1-4 Diagram representing different cross-sectional views of the femur, based on plane of section.

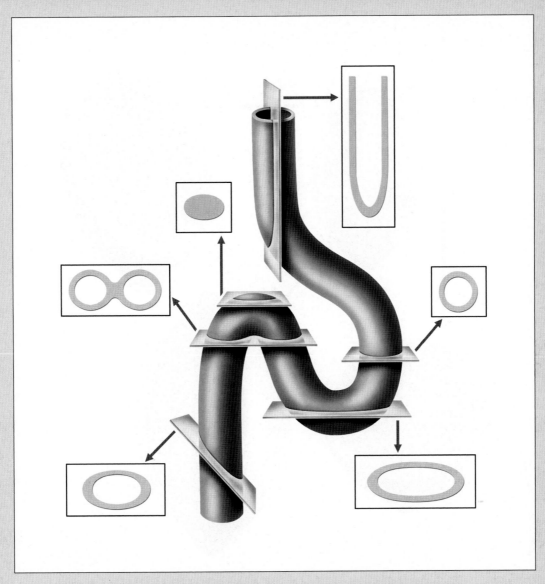

Figure 1-5 Diagram representing different sectional views of a hollow tube, based on plane of section.

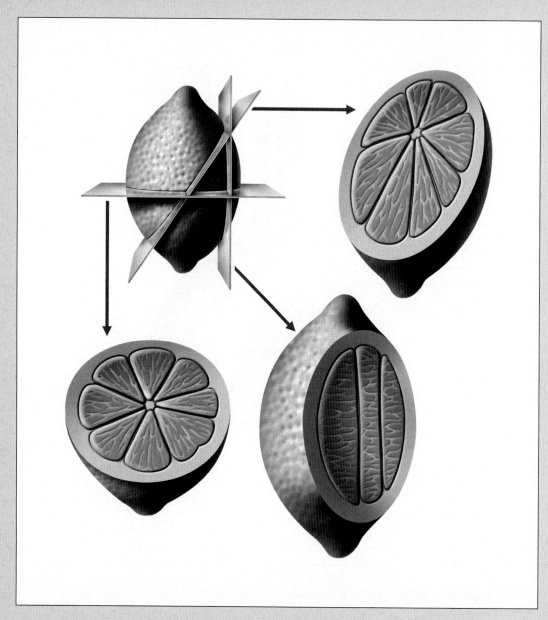

Figure 1-6 Diagram representing different sectional views of a lemon, based on plane of section.

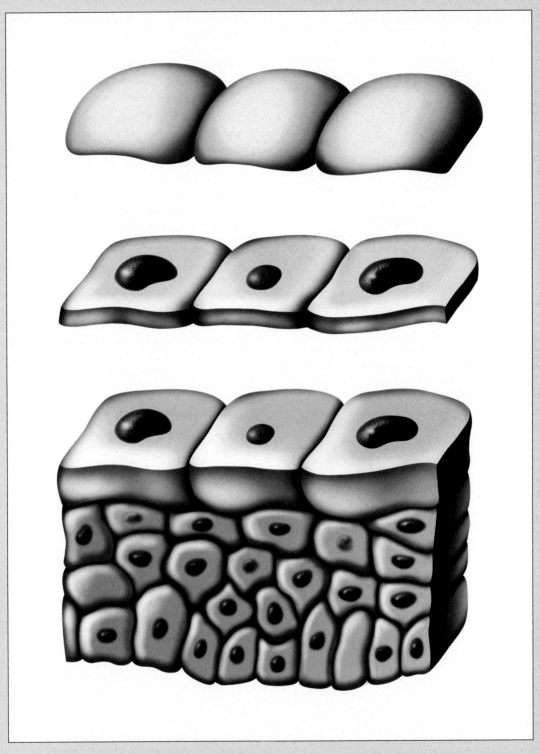

Figure 1-7 Diagram representing how the plane of section will alter the view of a tissue, depending on the level of sectioning.

Logic Trees—How to Develop Them

When you are attempting to identify an unknown epithelium or any other unknown slide, it is important to develop a methodology (such as the Logic Trees used in this book) that will yield reliable and correct results. Several things must be kept in mind as you learn how to develop your individual logic trees and progress through this book:

- To accurately identify unknown slides, one of the key skills that you must develop is the ability to ask simple, reliable "yes" or "no" questions in the proper order. Simply put, you want to obtain the most accurate answer in the shortest amount of time. Being able to identify a slide correctly by asking only three or four key questions will serve you better than correctly identifying a slide by following a "shotgun" approach and randomly asking questions in search of an answer.

- You should try to base an identification on a minimum of two or three characteristics. Artifacts—be they sectioning or staining—will crop up at the most inopportune times. As you progress through this book, note the artifacts in many of the photomicrographs. These have been included for a purpose—you need to become comfortable with artifacts and how they may affect your identification. Therefore, you should base every identification on no fewer than three reliable characteristics. Granted, there will be occasions when a correct identification may be made on fewer characteristics, and we will do our best to point out these instances to you.

- Do not memorize! As hard as it may be to fathom at this time, very little anatomy (gross or microscopic) is learned by memorization. You need to understand the three-dimensional anatomical characteristics of a specimen, as well as the relationships between structure and function, to fully grasp any branch of anatomy.

- Staining characteristics are important, but do not try to identify histological specimens solely on the basis of color. Although H & E is the most commonly used stain, you will encounter different stains as your study of histology progresses. If you memorized staining characteristics without understanding anatomical relationships, both three-dimensional and those of structure and function, you are almost guaranteed to identify an unknown preparation incorrectly.

- Remember to examine the specimen using multiple fields of view. Start examining every slide at the lowest power possible and then slowly progress to higher powers. Remember, you will make an accurate identification by looking at all of the tissue's characteristics, and the higher the viewing power the smaller the field of vision. Look at the entire specimen at each power and note the characteristics seen at each power.

REFERENCE

[1]Pugh MB, editor: *Stedman's Medical Dictionary*, ed 27, Baltimore, 2000, Lippincott Williams & Wilkins.

Chapter 2

EPITHELIAL TISSUE

Chapter Objectives

This chapter will enable you to:

1. Differentiate among the various cell shapes seen in epithelial tissue.

2. Differentiate among simple, stratified, pseudostratified, and transitional epithelia.

3. Understand the composition of a basal lamina.

4. Be able to identify goblet cells and mucous cells.

5. Understand the various types of glands formed by epithelial tissue.

Characteristics of Epithelial Tissue

Epithelial tissue is one of the four basic tissues of the body. The others are connective, muscular, and nervous tissue. Epithelial tissue lines all internal cavities and passageways of the human body and covers all exposed surfaces.

All epithelial tissues share the following common and important characteristics:

- Free surface: Epithelial tissue always has an apical surface or a free edge.

- Arranged into sheets or layers: All epithelial tissue is composed of a sheet of cells one or more layers thick.

- Cellularity: Epithelial tissue is composed almost entirely of cells bound closely together by specialized junctions. As a result, epithelial tissue has little or no intercellular space.

- Polarity: Because many epithelial tissues are involved in some form of cellular transport, epithelial tissue has polarity. In other words, epithelial cells have a distinct top and bottom, with cellular specializations and intracellular organelles arranged accordingly.

- Avascularity: Epithelial tissue lacks blood vessels. As a result, all cellular nutrients must be delivered and all cellular wastes must be removed via diffusion.

- Attachment: All epithelial tissues are firmly anchored to an underlying fibrous basal lamina that has been secreted by the overlying epithelium.

- Regeneration: Epithelial tissue is continually damaged or lost at the exposed internal and external surfaces of the body. These cells are continually replaced through mitosis of stem cells found within the epithelium.

Classification of Epithelial Tissues

Epithelial tissue is classified according to (1) the number of layers making up the epithelial sheet or gland, and (2) the shape of

the most superficial layer of these cells. Epithelial cells are categorized into one of the following three shapes:

- Squamous: When viewed from above, squamosal epithelial cells are described as appearing "scale-like" or like "sunny-side up" fried eggs. The thickness of the cytoplasm of these cells is usually too thin to be seen when viewed from the side with a light microscope. However, when the lateral cytoplasm can be seen, the nucleus of this cell type is often observed to bulge outward from the thin outline of the cell.

- Cuboidal: These cells are approximately equal in height and width. The nucleus of this cell type typically is positioned centrally within the cell.

- Columnar: This type of epithelial cell is taller than it is wide. The nucleus is usually located in the basal one third of the cell. However, some specialized columnar cells have an apically located nucleus.

As you examine the shapes of epithelial cells, note that the shape of the nucleus parallels that of the cell. In other words, the nuclei of squamous epithelial cells will often be attenuated and flattened, while those of cuboidal or columnar cells tend to be rounder.

In addition to cell shape, epithelial tissue is classified according to the number of layers present. Epithelial tissue may be:

- Simple: A single layer of epithelial cells in which all cells reach the underlying connective tissue (termed the *basal lamina*).

- Stratified: An epithelium composed of multiple layers of epithelial cells. In a stratified epithelium, only the cells of the basal layer reach the basal lamina, and only the most superficial layer of cells has a free surface.

- Pseudostratified: A single layer of epithelial cells in which the height of the cells varies considerably. In this type of epithelium, all cells reach the basal lamina, but not all cells reach the free surface. Because of the varying height of the cells and corresponding nucleus placement, the epithelium gives the appearance of being stratified.

- Transitional: This epithelium is characteristic of the urinary system. As the urinary tract organ stretches or relaxes, the cells of this epithelium will change shape, thereby giving the impression that the epithelium has changed from a multiple-layer to a single-layer arrangement.

Functions of Epithelial Tissue

Epithelial tissue serves a variety of functions, including secretion, absorption, and transport. In order to accomplish these functions, epithelial tissue will be found in the form of either sheets or glands. In addition, these sheets and glands will be composed of varying types of epithelial cells. In order to identify epithelial tissue, you must become familiar with the individual characteristics and components of the various types of epithelia. In this chapter, we will progress from identifying the varying cell shapes to identifying the layering of epithelial tissue. Finally, we will look at the processes used in the identification of the different types of epithelial cells.

Epithelial Sheets

Epithelial sheets are continuous sheets of cells that are joined by specialized intercellular junctions that cannot be seen with the light microscope. These sheets vary in thickness, ranging from one layer to multiple layers. The epithelial cells are attached to the underlying connective tissue by a basal lamina. A basal lamina is composed of two layers. (Neither of these sublayers of the basal lamina can be identified with the light microscope.) The most superficial layer of the basal lamina is called the *clear layer* (lamina lucida) and is secreted by the epithelial tissue. The deeper layer is the *dense layer* (lamina densa), secreted by the underlying connective tissue. The structural organization of the clear layer is dominated by large, coarse collagenous fibers, microfilaments, and glycoproteins; it serves as a diffusion barrier to proteins and other large macromolecules and contributes to the strength of the basal lamina.

Often the term *basement membrane* will be encountered in histological studies. In some multilayered epithelia, such as the stratified squamous epithelium of the skin, the basal lamina is anchored to underlying connective tissue by a series of anchoring collagenous fibrils. The proper use of the term *basement membrane* pertains only to the basal lamina and this layer of anchoring collagen fibers associated with some forms of multilayered epithelia.

Simple Epithelia

Simple Columnar Epithelium (Duodenum)

These photomicrographs are of a transverse section of the duodenum of the small intestine. First examine the specimen at low power (**Figure 2-1**) and then progress to higher magnifications.

The innermost layer of the small intestine is the mucosa, which is thrown into finger-like projections termed *villi*. These structures increase the absorptive and secretory surface area of the duodenum. The lumen of the organ is at the right of the figure. Note that the lumen appears to be filled with circular segments of villi. This is an excellent example of a *sectioning artifact*. As the intestinal villi twist and turn, the plane of section will vary from longitudinal sections to cross sections—hence the varied appearance of the villi seen in this section.

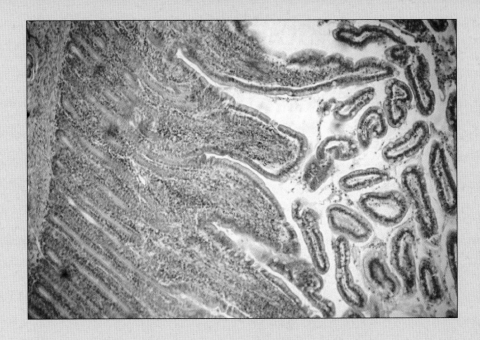

Villus

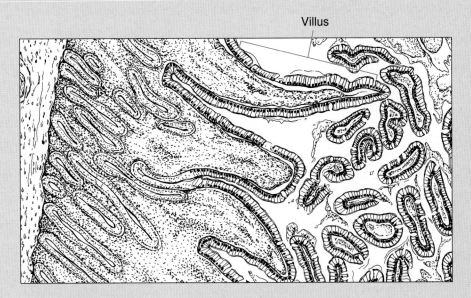

Figure 2-1 (25×): Villi of the duodenum of the small intestine.

As you progress from low to medium (Figure 2-2) to high-dry (Figure 2-3), note that the epithelial layer on the villi is a *simple columnar epithelium*. The tissue beneath the epithelium contains a variety of cell types, the nuclei of which give the region a granular appearance at low power.

As you examine the simple columnar epithelium, note the following:

• These cells are taller than wide, and all of the basal surfaces of the cells contact the *basal lamina*.

• The *nucleus* of this type of epithelium is typically found in the basal one third of the cell. In addition, the nuclei of a simple columnar epithelium are arranged in such a way that they are all at approximately the same level.

Note the presence of a fixation artifact in these two photomicrographs. This artifact is due to shrinkage of the specimen during fixation and gives the appearance that the epithelium is pulled away from the underlying connective tissue.

Figure 2-3 is a photomicrograph taken using the high-dry objective. Note the dark line at the free surface of the epithelium. This represents a cellular modification, termed the *microvillus border*, which serves to increase the surface area of the cell's apical surface.

The *basal lamina*, although difficult to see, is visible as a thin, fibrous line at the base of the cells. Do not confuse it with the elongated cells in the tissue deep to the epithelium.

Throughout the epithelium you see small spherical or flask-shaped "holes." These spaces are actually unicellular glands, termed *goblet cells*. Goblet cells secrete a substance termed *mucinogen*. Goblet cells have a clear or hollow appearance as a result of the dissolution of mucinogen during the histological processing.

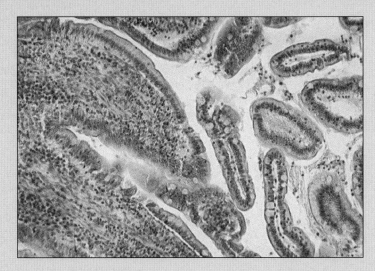

Figure 2-2 (50×): Simple columnar epithelium of duodenal villi.

Figure 2-3 (100×): Simple columnar epithelium of duodenal villi.

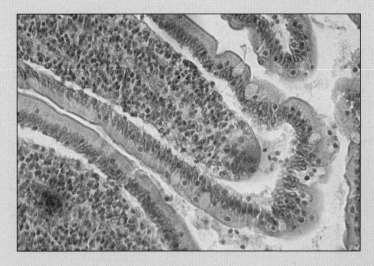

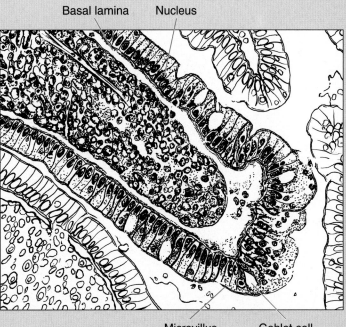

Basal lamina   Nucleus

Microvillus border   Goblet cell

Simple Cuboidal and Simple Squamous Epithelia (Renal Medulla)

Figures 2-4 and 2-5 were taken from the medulla of the kidney. The medullary region of the kidney is composed of a large number of tubules: descending limbs of the proximal convoluted tubule, nephron loops (loops of Henle), and the ascending limbs of the distal convoluted tubules. The vasa recta of the renal vasculature is also present within the medulla. All of these structures have a *simple epithelium*, ranging from *simple squamous* to *simple cuboidal*. As discussed earlier (see Classification of Epithelial Tissues), simple cuboidal epithelial cells are approximately equal in height and width. A simple squamous epithelium, in contrast, is composed of attenuated cells, the nucleus of which often bulges outward from the thin outline of the cell.

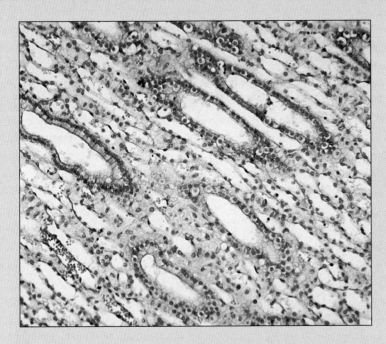

Figure 2-4 (50×): Simple cuboidal and simple squamous epithelium of the renal medulla.

Figure 2-5 (100×): Simple cuboidal and simple squamous epithelium of the renal medulla.

Simple cuboidal epithelium

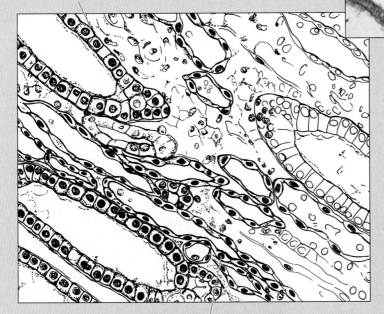

Simple squamous epithelium

Stratified Epithelia

A stratified epithelium is composed of two or more layers of epithelial cells. The cells of the uppermost layer of a stratified epithelium do not reach the basal lamina but do reach the luminal surface. In contrast, those of the lowest layer do not reach the surface but do contact the underlying basal lamina. *The classification of a stratified epithelium is based only on the appearance of the most superficial layer of cells.*

Stratified Squamous Epithelium (Mucosal Type) (Esophagus)

Nonkeratinized, stratified squamous epithelium (mucosal type) is found on structures of the body that are moist and subjected to significant abrasion, such as those found in the esophagus and vaginal cavity. These photomicrographs demonstrate the non-keratinized, stratified squamous epithelium (mucosal type) found in the esophagus.

As you progress from low power (Figure 2-6), to medium power (Figure 2-7), and finally to high-dry (Figure 2-8), you will note the following in these photomicrographs:

- The epithelium is composed of multiple layers, thereby making it a stratified epithelium.

- The nuclei of the cells in this epithelium appear to be "regularly arranged;" that is, they *appear* to be arranged into distinct layers.

- Although the cells of the deepest layers of the epithelium are cuboidal in shape, the superficial layer of cells is composed of squamous cells, thereby classifying this epithelium as stratified squamous.

Deep to the epithelium are the *basal lamina* and a loose layer of connective tissue, termed the *lamina propria*, which may or may not be visible in your preparation.

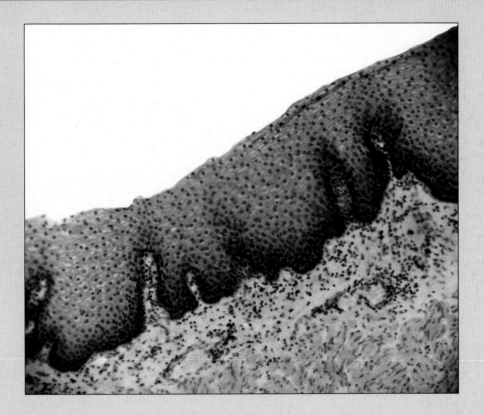

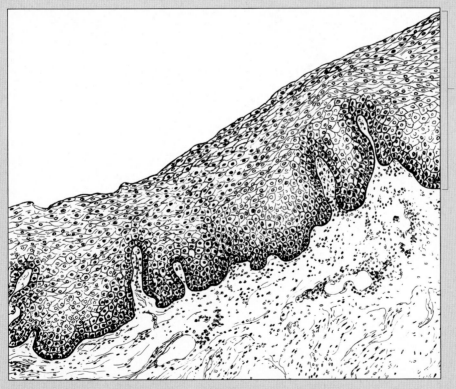

Stratified
epithelium

Figure 2-6 (25×): Stratified squamous epithelium of the esophagus.

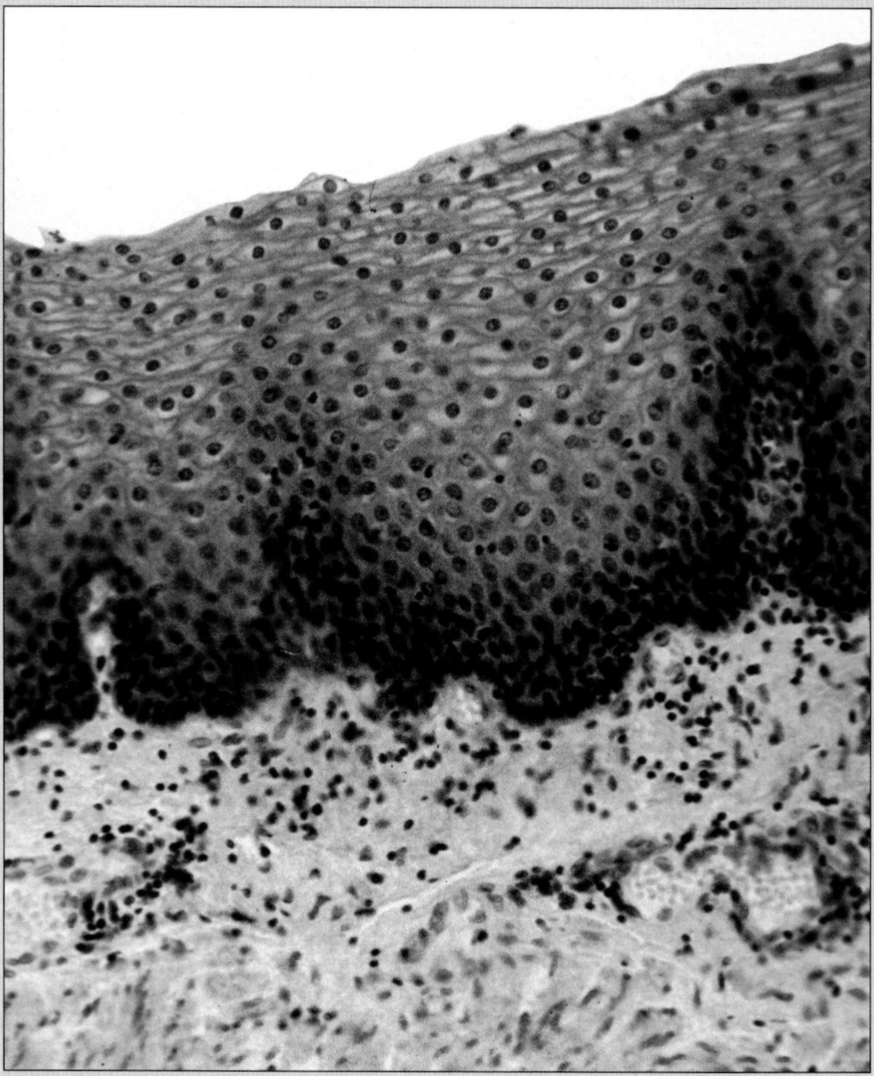

Figure 2-7 (50×): Stratified squamous epithelium of the esophagus.

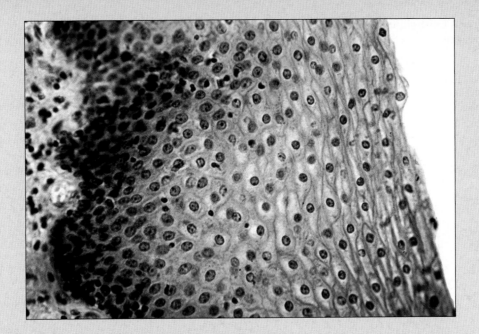

Stratified epithelium

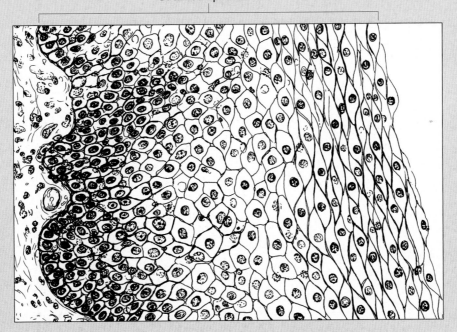

Figure 2-8 (100×): Stratified squamous epithelium of the esophagus.

Stratified Squamous Epithelium (Keratinized) (Thin Skin/Caucasian)

Figures 2-9 and 2-10 were obtained from thin Caucasian skin. This type of epithelium is found on surfaces of the body that are subjected to significant abrasion. Note the sectioning and preparation artifacts in this slide.

As you compare Figures 2-9 and 2-10 with those examined previously (see Figures 2-6 to 2-8), you will note some subtle similarities and differences between these two examples of stratified squamous epithelium:

- The epithelium in all of the figures is composed of multiple layers, thereby making it a stratified epithelium.

- The nuclei of the cells in this epithelium appear to be "regularly arranged;" that is, they appear to be arranged into distinct layers. However, this is significantly more apparent in Figures 2-6 through 2-8 than in Figures 2-9 and 2-10.

- Although the basal cells are cuboidal in shape, the superficial layer of cells in both of these epithelia is composed of squamosal cells.

Examination of Figures 2-9 and 2-10 demonstrates that the most superficial layer of this epithelium is composed of a *keratinized layer.* This layer is composed of dead, anucleated squamous cells that are continuously being sloughed off. These cells give the protective characteristics to the skin.

Again, remember that the classification of a stratified epithelium is based on the shape of the most superficial layer of cells—hence this epithelium is classified as a stratified squamous epithelium.

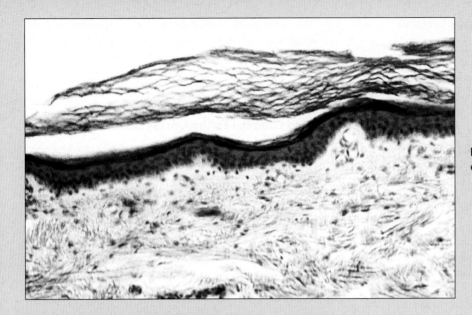

Figure 2-9 (50×): Stratified squamous epithelium (thin skin/Caucasian).

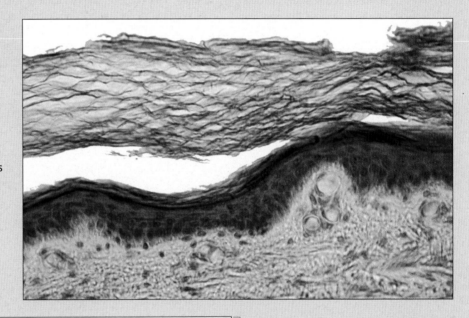

Figure 2-10 (100×): Stratified squamous epithelium (thin skin/Caucasian).

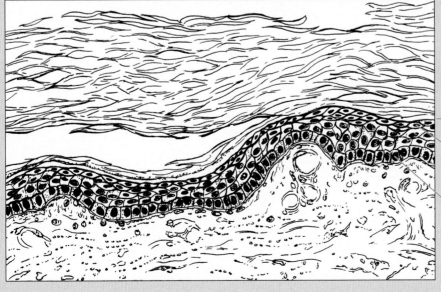

Keratinized layer

Squamosal-shaped cells

Cuboidal-shaped cells

Stratified Columnar Epithelium (Spongy Urethra)

Figure 2-11 is of the spongy (cavernous or penile) portion of the male urethra and shows an epithelium composed of several layers. The most superficial layer of this epithelium is composed of columnar epithelial cells.

Note the following:

- This is an epithelium composed of more than one layer, and therefore it is classified as a stratified epithelium.

- The nuclei of the epithelial cells appear to be arranged into rows, again suggesting a stratified epithelium.

- The cells in the superficial layer are taller than they are wide, indicating a columnar epithelium.

Each of the cells in the superficial layer has its nucleus in the basal portion of the cell, again indicating a columnar epithelium. *All of these are important histological characteristics of a stratified columnar epithelium.*

Finally, note how the depth of the epithelium, as well as the overall focus of the structure, varies within the specimen. This is an excellent example of how the appearance of an epithelium may vary from place to place because of a *sectioning artifact.* The appearance of a sectioning artifact in this photomicrograph, and the way in which the image fades from in focus to out of focus, clearly indicates the need to look at the entire specimen before categorizing the epithelium.

Stratified Cuboidal Epithelium (Sweat Gland Duct)

A stratified cuboidal epithelium (Figure 2-12) is characterized by two or more layers of cells, with a superficial layer of *cuboidal-shaped cells.*

Although the lateral borders of the superficial cells are not clearly evident, several characteristics indicate that these cells are indeed cuboidal:

- The nucleus is located within the central portion of the cell.

- The apical cells are approximately equal in height and width.

These characteristics, when taken together, indicate that this epithelium is stratified cuboidal.

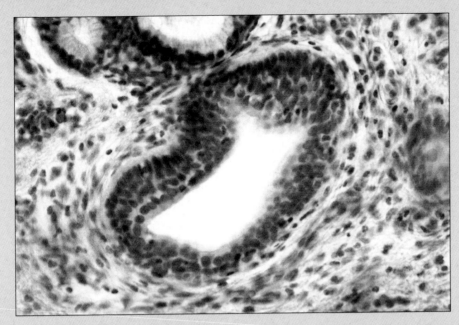

Figure 2-11 (100×): Stratified columnar epithelium (cavernous urethra).

Figure 2-12 (100×): Stratified cuboidal epithelium (sweat gland duct).

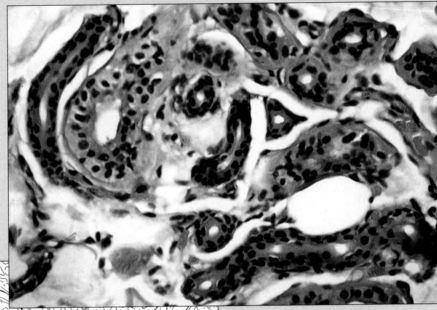

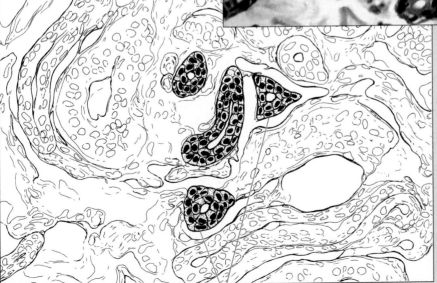

Ducts with stratified cuboidal epithelium

Pseudostratified Epithelia

Pseudostratified Ciliated Columnar Epithelium (Trachea)

These photomicrographs were taken from the trachea. As you look at Figure 2-13, note the epithelium and its characteristics. *Note that the epithelial nuclei are at varying levels*, thereby giving the appearance of an epithelium composed of several layers.

Now proceed to Figure 2-14. *Note that the nuclei appear to be randomly arranged within the epithelium; this is a key characteristic of a pseudostratified epithelium.* Continued examination demonstrates that the cells, even though they may be of different heights, are all considerably taller than they are wide, a feature that is characteristic of a columnar epithelium.

Although it cannot be demonstrated with the light microscope, all of the cells of this epithelium *do indeed reach the basal lamina but vary considerably in height*. Because all of the cells reach the underlying basal lamina, this epithelium cannot be classified as stratified. In addition, because of the variation in the height of the cells, not all of the cells reach the luminal surface. This variation in cell height and the corresponding nucleus location contribute to the appearance of a stratified epithelium—hence the designation of a *pseudostratified epithelium;* that is, an epithelium that has the appearance of being stratified but is not.

The apical surface of the cells in Figure 2-14 demonstrates a surface modification commonly seen in epithelial cells—*cilia.*

Also visible in Figure 2-14 are a few *mucous cells,* which are commonly seen in the pseudostratified columnar epithelium of the trachea.

Finally, this epithelium sits on an unusually thick *basal lamina.* The gap seen between the epithelium and the underlying basal lamina in this photomicrograph is a *fixation artifact.*

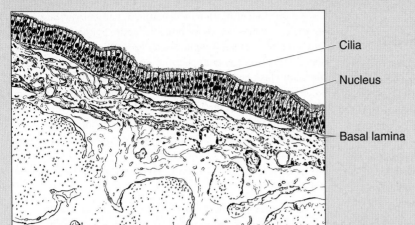

Cilia

Nucleus

Basal lamina

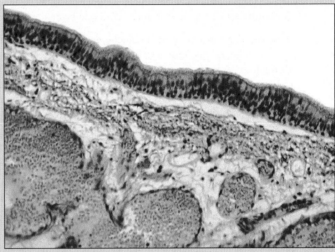

Figure 2-13 (50×): Pseudostratified ciliated columnar epithelium (trachea).

Mucous cell

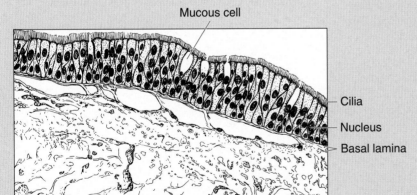

Cilia

Nucleus

Basal lamina

Figure 2-14 (100×): Pseudostratified ciliated columnar epithelium (trachea).

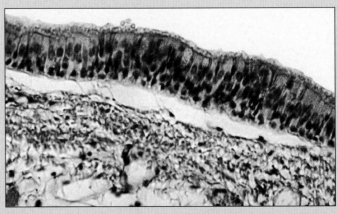

Transitional Epithelia

Transitional Epithelium (Relaxed Urinary Bladder)

The distribution of this epithelium is limited to the urinary tract. The appearance of the cells that comprise this type of epithelium will vary depending on the state of stretch of the organ at the time of fixation; hence the name *transitional.* Because of this inherent variability, transitional epithelium is one of the most difficult epithelia to identify correctly.

The cells at the free surface of a transitional epithelium are described as dome shaped, or balloon shaped, broadly cuboidal, or somewhat flattened (approaching squamous), depending on the state of stretch of the organ. Examination of Figure 2-15 will show the following:

- An epithelium composed of more than one layer

- A "regular" arrangement of the nuclei, in that the nuclei appear to be arranged in rows (as seen in Figures 2-7 through 2-12, but not in Figure 2-13)

- A variation in cell shape when you compare the deepest layer with the most superficial layer

- Cells at the free surface that typically are large and rounded (characteristic of a relaxed organ) or flattened, almost squamous in shape (characteristic of a stretched and distended organ)

- If the surface layer is squamous in shape, an abrupt change will be seen in cell shape from the superficial layer to deeper layers, where the cells will be larger and more rounded

These characteristics might lead you to incorrectly identify this epithelium as a stratified epithelium—possibly a stratified cuboidal or stratified columnar epithelium, or even a stratified squamous epithelium. However, further examination will lead you to a correct identification of this epithelium.

A correct identification of all epithelia, particularly transitional epithelia, requires you to examine the entire epithelial surface—a process often termed *running the epithelium.* In order to correctly identify transitional epithelium, you must slowly run the epithelium. This is accomplished by slowly scanning the entire epithelium from one end of the specimen to the other. Start at the end of the epithelium in the lower right side of the photomicrograph (see Figure 2-15). Now proceed toward the middle of the photomicrograph and then continue until you complete your examination at the other end of the epithelium. As you run the epithelium, additional characteristics of a relaxed transitional epithelium come to light:

- *The shape of the most superficial cells on this specimen changes from region to region.* If you run the epithelium from the lower right of Figure 2-15, you will note that the most superficial layer of cells ranges from almost squamous to something approaching cuboidal, and finally to a series of rounded or dome-shaped cells. As you approach the upper left corner of the epithelium, the cell shape again approaches squamous. *This variation in the shape of the most superficial layer of cells is an important identification feature of a relaxed transitional epithelium.*

- *The number of layers in the epithelium appears to vary from region to region.* This, too, is an important identification feature of a relaxed transitional epithelium.

- When transitional epithelium is obtained from a relaxed organ, the surface cells often bulge into the lumen (often referred to as *dome- or balloon-shaped* cells), another important identification feature of transitional epithelium.

- This photomicrograph also demonstrates that transitional epithelia may have binuclear cells on the apical surface.

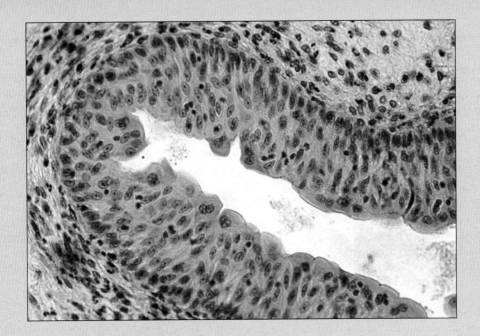

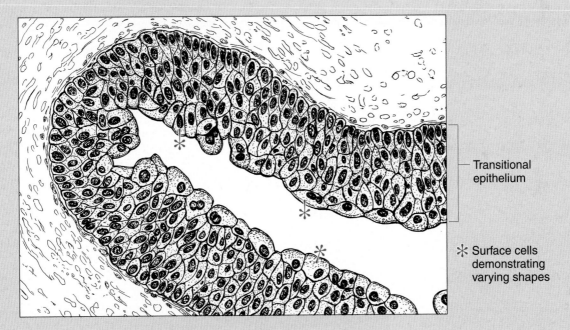

Figure 2-15 (100×): Transitional epithelium (relaxed urinary bladder).

Transitional epithelium

＊ Surface cells demonstrating varying shapes

Epithelial Glands

Epithelial glands are the second main form of epithelial tissue. Epithelial glands are classified as either endocrine glands or exocrine glands.

Endocrine glands are ductless glands that release their secretions directly onto the cell's surface or directly into the lymphoid system, interstitial fluids, or bloodstream.

Exocrine glands are those that possess ducts or that deliver their secretion to an apical or luminal surface. These glands may be either unicellular (e.g., goblet cells and mucous cells) or multicellular. Multicellular exocrine glands are composed of two parts: a secretory portion and a duct that conveys the secretion to the epithelial surface. Multicellular exocrine glands are typically subdivided by the structure of their ducts. Simple exocrine glands possess an unbranched duct, whereas a compound exocrine gland possesses a duct that branches repeatedly.

Compound exocrine glands may be further subdivided based on the shape of the secretory portion of the gland. An acinar gland is a compound exocrine gland, the secretory portion of which is flask shaped; the secretory portion of a tubular gland is shaped like a tube. Some glands (e.g., mammary glands and the pancreas) may be a combination of a tubular and acinar gland. Such glands would then be classified as tubuloacinar glands.

Exocrine Glands

Unicellular Exocrine Glands

Figures 2-3 and 2-14 demonstrate unicellular exocrine glands. *Goblet cells* (see Figure 2-3) are commonly found within many regions of the digestive tract, whereas *mucous cells* (see Figure 2-14) are found within portions of the respiratory tree. Goblet and mucous cells often give the appearance of being clear or empty. They have this appearance as a result of the dissolution of the mucinogen during histological processing.

Simple Glands (Sweat Glands)

Sweat glands are multicellular glands that possess a distal secretory portion in which the epithelial cells produce the secretion, and an epithelial duct that carries the secretion to the exterior of the gland. Although the distal secretory portion is not visible in this section, Figure 2-16 demonstrates how the duct is repeatedly sectioned into circular segments because of the convoluted shape of the tubular portion of the gland. Note that the duct does not appear to go to the surface. This is the result of the plane of section and illustrates how you must keep the three-dimensional organization of a structure in mind when viewing histological preparations.

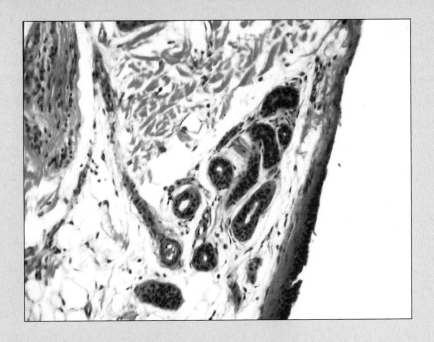

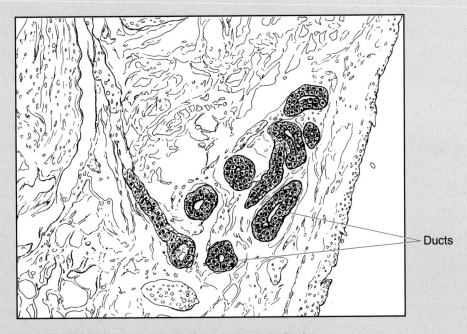

Ducts

Figure 2-16 (100×): Simple epithelial glands (sweat glands).

Simple Glands (Intestinal Crypts)

Figure 2-17 demonstrates *unbranched, simple tubular exocrine glands of the duodenum of the small intestine* (called *intestinal crypts*). These simple glands are formed by the surface epithe-lium extending deep into the mucosal layer of the duodenum, thereby forming a straight tubule that opens directly onto the epithelial surface via a simple, unbranched duct.

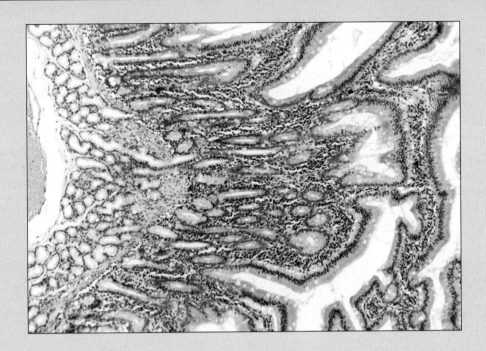

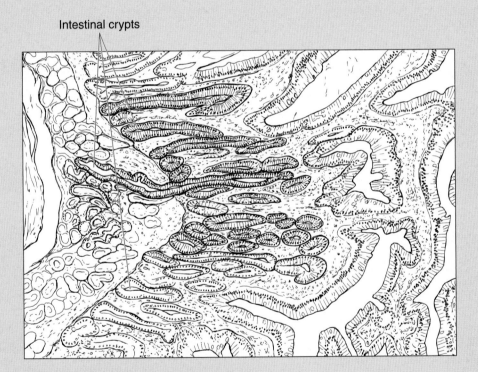

Intestinal crypts

Figure 2-17 (50×): Simple glands (duodenum).

Compound Tubuloacinar Glands

Mammary Gland

The mammary gland (Figure 2-18) is composed of secretory acini and excretory ducts and is therefore a compound tubuloacinar gland.

Parotid Salivary Gland

The parotid salivary gland (Figure 2-19) is another excellent example of a compound tubuloacinar gland. For this slide, concentrate on the shape and composition of an acinar gland. Later (see Chapter 16) you will learn about the histological charac-teristics that will enable you to correctly identify the different types of salivary glands.

Acinar glands are epithelial glands that contain circular or flask-shaped secretory segments. In this slide, note both the *secretory acini* and *ducts* of the salivary gland. One way to visu-alize an acinus is to imagine an orange or grapefruit that has been cut into a cross section (see Figure 1-3). Each wedge of the fruit represents a columnar acinar cell. This cell shape is termed *columnar* because the cell is taller than it is wide. The central portion of the fruit section is the *centroacinar duct* of the gland, and the skin of the fruit represents the *basal lamina* of the glandular acinus.

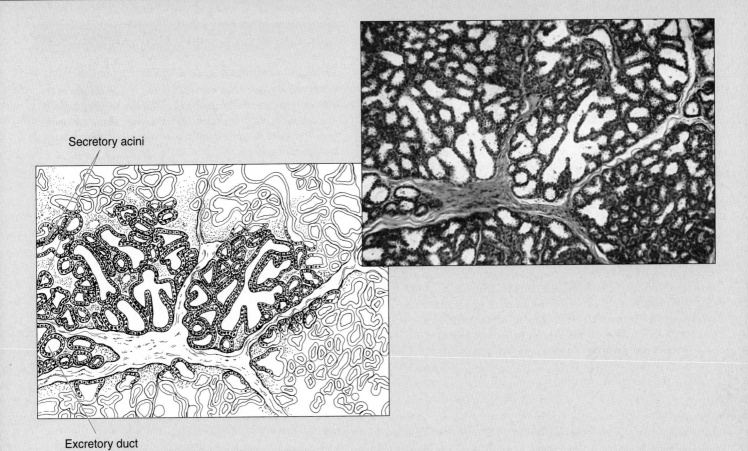

Secretory acini

Excretory duct

Figure 2-18 (100×): Compound tubuloacinar epithelial glands (mammary gland).

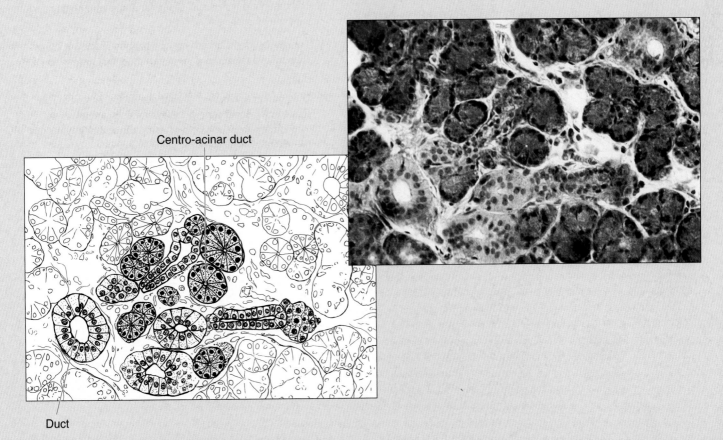

Centro-acinar duct

Duct

Figure 2-19 (200×): Compound tubuloacinar gland (parotid salivary gland).

Endocrine Glands

A complete histological explanation of endocrine glands is provided in Chapter 14.

Endocrine Pancreas (Pancreatic Islets, or Islets of Langerhans)

Figure 2-20 is a high-dry photomicrograph of *pancreatic islets* (Islets of Langerhans), which comprise the endocrine portion of the pancreas. Endocrine glands are often composed of *epithelioid* cells; that is, cells that are predominantly derived from epithelial tissue and therefore have epithelial characteristics. (An exception to this rule is the neurohypophysis, or posterior lobe of the pituitary gland, which is derived from neural tissue.) Their secretions are released into the vascular system without the use of ducts. Endocrine glands may be unicellular, such as the enteroendocrine cells within the digestive system, or multicellular, such as the endocrine portion of the pancreas. If an endocrine gland is multicellular, the cells may be grouped together into an organ, such as the thyroid gland, or may be scattered throughout an organ, as are the islets of the pancreas.

Commonly Misidentified Tissues

Stratified Squamous and Transitional Epithelia

When you are looking at epithelial tissue, it is important to remember that stratified squamous epithelium (nonkeratinized, mucosal type) and transitional epithelium are easily misidentified. Therefore keep in mind the differences between these two types of epithelium.

Stratified Squamous Epithelium (Nonkeratinized, Mucosal Type) (Review **Figures 2-6** to **2-8** in "Stratified Epithelia" section, pp. 20–23)

1. Stratified squamous epithelium is composed of many layers.

2. The basal cells may appear to be cuboidal or columnar in shape.

3. The surface layer is always composed of flattened cells.

4. The number and extent of epithelial layers, as well as the shape of the most superficial layer of cells, are relatively consistent from one field of vision to another as you "run the epithelium."

Transitional Epithelium (Review **Figure 2-15** in "Transitional Epithelia" section, pp. 28, 30–31)

1. Transitional epithelium has fewer layers in comparison with stratified squamous epithelium.

2. The basal cells are usually of similar shape when compared with the most superficial cells.

3. The most superficial cells may be balloon shaped or dome shaped (in a relaxed organ) or flattened (in a distended organ).

4. The number and extent of epithelial layers, as well as the shape of the most superficial layer of cells, are relatively inconsistent from one field of vision to another as you "run the epithelium."

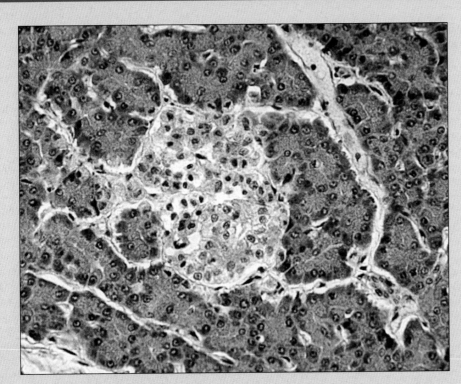

Figure 2-20 (200×): Endocrine pancreas (Islets of Langerhans).

Logic Tree

LOGIC TREE FOR EPITHELIUM

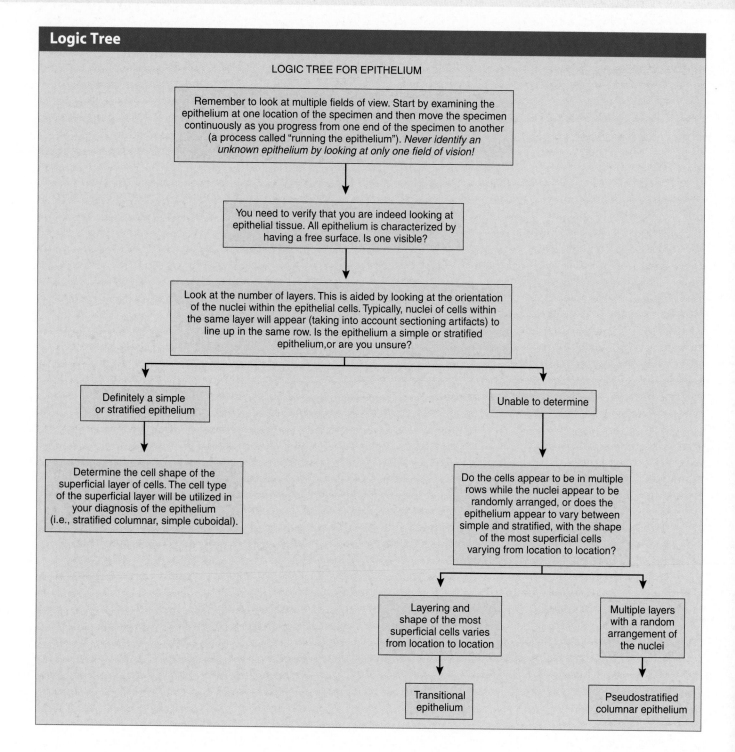

Chapter 3

CONNECTIVE TISSUE PROPER

Chapter Objectives

This chapter will enable you to:

1. Differentiate among the subclasses of connective tissue discussed in this chapter, including:

   - Loose, irregular (areolar) connective tissue

   - White (unilocular) and brown (multilocular) fat

   - Reticular connective tissue

   - Dense irregular connective tissue

   - Dense regular connective tissue, including tendon and elastic (yellow) ligament

2. Identify the different cells and fiber types found in connective tissue

Connective Tissue Function and Composition

Connective tissue is subdivided into the following categories and subcategories:

- Connective Tissue Proper

  - Loose connective tissue proper

    —Loose, irregular (areolar) connective tissue

    —White and brown fat*

    —Reticular connective tissue

  - Dense connective tissue proper

    —Irregular dense connective tissue

    —Regular dense connective tissue (tendons and ligaments)

- Specialized Connective Tissue

  - Cartilage

  - Bone

  - Blood

Functions of Connective Tissue

All forms of connective tissue perform a variety of functions, including:

- Filler and packer, in that the body has few, if any "empty" spaces within it

- Energy storage

- Ion storage

- Support

- Protection

- Attachment

- Insulation

- Serving as a diffusion medium for the transport of oxygen, carbon dioxide, and nutrients

Connective tissue is composed of cells and an extracellular matrix. The extracellular matrix is, in turn, composed of a ground substance and organic connective tissue fibers that provide support and attachment. The ground substance consists of structural glycoproteins, proteoglycans, electrolytes, and other

---

*White and brown fat are considered to be a form of specialized connective tissue by some histologists.

components that serve as a diffusion medium and also provide varying amounts of support. The proportions of these two components (fibers and ground substance), as well as their composition, will vary from one type of connective tissue to another. The extracellular matrix will also vary in consistency from one form of connective tissue to another. *Indeed, connective tissues, with the exception of adipose tissue, are identified by the histological characteristics of the extracellular matrix.*

Connective tissue, with some exceptions, generally has a rich blood supply, thereby allowing it to provide nutrients to adjacent tissues.

Loose, Irregular (Areolar) Connective Tissue

Loose, irregular connective tissue (also termed *loose areolar connective tissue*) derives its name from the arrangement of its intercellular fibers and the way in which they divide the extracellular matrix into small spaces (areola). The fibers of loose, irregular connective tissue are loosely and irregularly arranged, thereby making the diagnosis of cell and fiber types relatively easy.

This type of connective tissue is distributed widely throughout the body. It is found in the following anatomical locations:

- Surrounding blood vessels and nerves

- Forming superficial and deep subcutaneous fascia, mesenteries, and a portion of the supporting framework for most of the organs of the body

- Filling open spaces and cavities throughout the body

Loose, irregular connective tissue contains a varying population of fixed and wandering cells, including fibroblasts, fibrocytes, adipose cells (adipocytes or fat cells), mast cells, plasmocytes (plasma cells), and macrophages. If the number of adipose cells is high, then the tissue is appropriately named *adipose tissue*. Loose, irregular connective tissue will regularly contain all three possible fiber types: collagen, reticular, and elastic fibers.

Loose, Irregular Connective Tissue (Mesenteric Spread)

Figures 3-1 and 3-2 show a mesenteric spread. The best way to identify collagen, reticular, and elastic fibers within tissue preparations is via the use of specialized stains (see Appendix). *Collagen, reticular,* and *elastic fibers* may be seen within these photomicrographs.

- *Collagen fibers* are the dominant fiber type within loose, irregular connective tissue. Collagen fibers appear as wide, wavy, ribbon-like bands that stain with acidic dyes, such as eosin. These fibers will have varying diameters and may appear longitudinally striated because of their fibrillar substructure.

- *Elastic fibers* are considerably thinner than collagenous fibers and typically appear as straight, narrow, single fibers that branch frequently. Even though elastic fibers do not typically stain in standard hematoxylin and eosin (H & E) preparations, they may be seen within these photomicrographs because of their high degree of refractive ability (refringence).

- *Reticular fibers* are present in varying numbers in loose, irregular connective tissue. These fibers constitute the support network of many anatomical structures. Reticular fibers are narrow bundles of collagen fibrils that are coated with glycoproteins and proteoglycans, resulting in special staining properties. Specific stains must be used to see reticular fibers, and therefore they may not be seen within H & E photomicrographs. Reticular fibers are quite fine and branch frequently because of the longitudinal splitting of the collagen bundles.

The cellular population within loose, irregular connective tissue will vary considerably from one preparation to another. This variation will depend on the immunological status of the person or animal from which the preparation was obtained. **Figures 3-1** and **3-2** demonstrate *fibrocytes, macrophages,* and *mast cells.*

- *Fibrocytes* are the most numerous cells within loose, irregular connective tissue. They are responsible for maintaining the fibers within the extracellular matrix, as compared with fibroblasts, which secrete the connective tissue fibers. Therefore fibrocytes are minimally involved in the secretion of proteins. As a result, the cytoplasm of fibrocytes will stain clear to lightly acidophilic and will be poorly visible in H & E preparations.

- *Macrophages* are the second most common cell type of loose, irregular connective tissue. Macrophages are irregularly shaped cells with a rounded, dark staining nucleus. Inactive macrophages are difficult to distinguish from fibrocytes with the light microscope.

- *Mast cells* are some of the largest wandering cells of connective tissue. They occur in varying numbers within loose, irregular connective tissue but are especially numerous around blood vessels and deep to the epithelium of the respiratory and gastrointestinal systems. Mast cells are large cells with ovoid nuclei and possess numerous cytoplasmic granules that are basophilic. However, these granules are water soluble and therefore may be difficult to see in H & E preparations.

Loose, Irregular Connective Tissue (Lamina Propria of the Duodenum)

Figure 3-3 is a high-dry photomicrograph of the loose connective tissue normally found within the lamina propria of the duodenum. This layer of connective tissue is typically highly vascular and contains a varying population of fixed and wandering connective tissue cells. **Figure 3-3** demonstrates a variety of connective tissue cells, including *fibrocytes* and *plasmocytes (plasma cells).*

Plasmocytes are relatively rare in loose, irregular connective tissue under normal circumstances, but their numbers increase considerably during the inflammation process. Plasmocytes are small and irregularly shaped cells, with a relatively small and eccentrically placed nucleus. *The nuclear chromatin appears as deep staining granules arranged in such a way as to give the cell a "clock-faced" appearance, which is a major histological feature of this cell type.*

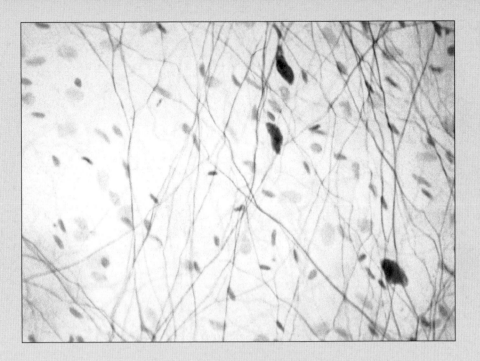

Reticular fiber

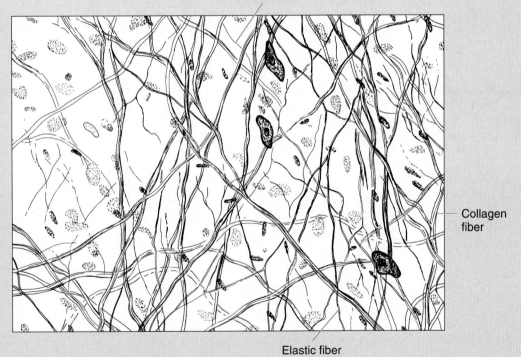

Collagen
fiber

Elastic fiber

Figure 3-1 (50×): Loose, irregular connective tissue (mesenteric spread).

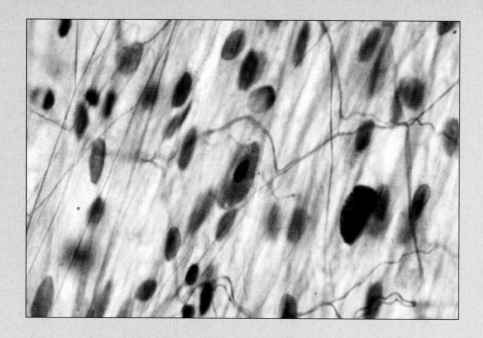

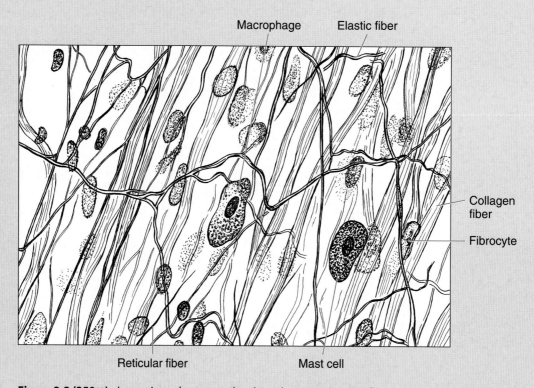

Figure 3-2 (250×): Loose, irregular connective tissue (mesenteric spread).

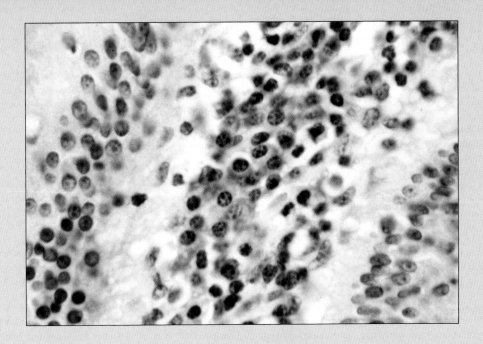

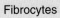 Fibrocytes

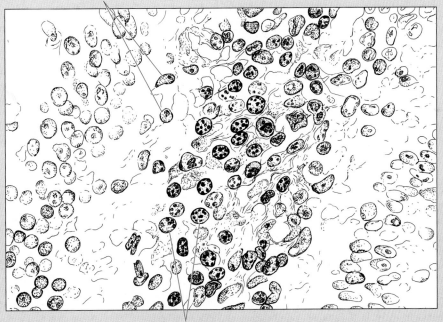

Plasmocytes

Figure 3-3 (100×): Loose, irregular connective tissue (lamina propria of duodenum).

Adipose Tissue

Adipose cells (adipocytes) are found singly or in groups in almost all forms of loose, irregular connective tissue. In certain anatomical locations, however, adipose cells will be found in high numbers and will be organized in such a way that the resulting tissue is designated as adipose tissue. When arranged into adipose tissue, adipose cells are regarded as fixed connective tissue cells.

Adipose tissue differs from other forms of connective tissue in that the intercellular material does not make up the bulk of the tissue. As a result, it is not used as the main histological characteristic for this tissue. In contrast, the cells and their contents are the main histological features of adipose tissue.

Adipose tissue may be subdivided into white (unilocular) and brown (multilocular) adipose tissue (fat). This subdivision is based on the color of the fat when viewed on gross dissection, as well as the method by which the cells store the fat globules.

White (Unilocular) Adipose Tissue

Figure 3-4 is a photomicrograph of white (unilocular) adipose tissue taken from the connective tissue surrounding the pancreas. This photomicrograph presents typical white adipose cells (unilocular adipocytes), as well as numerous cells that were damaged during sectioning and preservation, an artifact commonly seen in such histological preparations.

The following are characteristics of adipose cells of white fat:

- Individual fat droplets fuse to form a large, single fat droplet that comes to occupy the greater proportion of the cell.

- The *nucleus* is forced to the periphery of the cell. The cytoplasm becomes quite attenuated and forms a thin peripheral layer within the cell. It is because of this position of the nucleus and the small amount of cytoplasm that white adipose cells are described as having a "signet ring" conformation.

- Adipose cells have a clear or hollow appearance as a result of the dissolution of the fat droplet during the histological processing, thus leaving an empty space within the cell.

Adipose tissue differs from other forms of connective tissue in that individual adipose cells are surrounded by a thin basal lamina that may or may not be visible in light microscope sections. In addition, adipose tissue is highly vascularized, and a large number of *capillaries* are visible within this section.

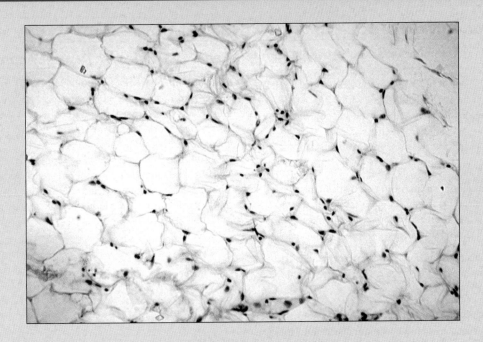

Capillary   Nucleus   Capillary

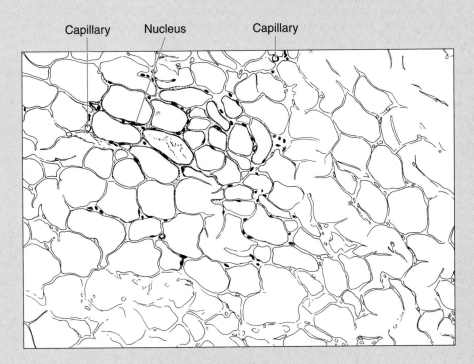

Figure 3-4 (50×): White (unilocular) adipose tissue.

Brown (Multilocular) Adipose Tissue

Figure 3-5 demonstrates brown (multilocular) fat intermixed with white fat. Brown fat has a widespread distribution in hibernating animals, whereas in humans it has a considerably smaller distribution. Brown fat is typically found within the interscapular and inguinal regions of humans, with the amount decreasing after birth.

Brown fat differs from white fat (Figure 3-4) in the following two ways:

- White fat stores all of the lipid droplets within one coalesced lipid droplet, whereas brown fat stores the lipid droplets within multiple cytoplasmic vacuoles—hence the multilocular appearance of brown adipose cells.

- As a result of this form of lipid storage in brown fat, the nucleus is typically centrally located within the cell and is round in shape.

Also visible within this photomicrograph are several connective tissue septa, which divide the adipose tissue into lobules. Some of the septa have blood vessels associated with them.

Reticular Connective Tissue

Reticular Connective Tissue (Lymph Node)

Reticular fibers are not visible in routine H & E sections. A particular stain called *reticulin stain* (see Appendix) must be used to see this fiber type. Reticular connective tissue forms a structural framework for many tissues and organs, including bone marrow and lymphoid organs.

In Figure 3-6, *reticular fibers* appear dark blue to black and obscure the underlying lymphoid cells. As you examine this photomicrograph, note that the reticular fibers may be found singly or in clumps. Single fibers have a relatively thin diameter and branch considerably.

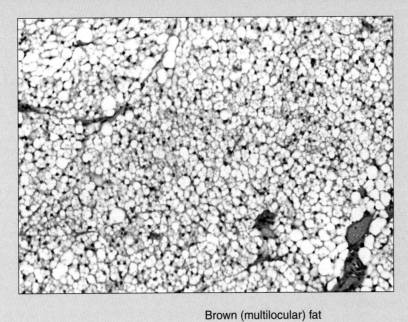

Figure 3-5 (50×): Brown (multilocular) adipose tissue.

Brown (multilocular) fat

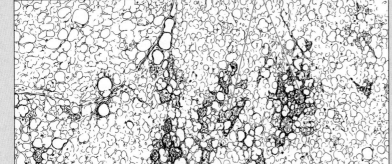

Figure 3-6 (50×): Reticular connective tissue (lymph node).

Dense Irregular Connective Tissue

Dense irregular connective tissue differs from loose, irregular connective tissue in the following ways:

- The connective tissue fibers within the extracellular matrix are more densely arranged because of the higher concentration of thick bundles of collagen fibers.

- The cells are fewer in number and type. Dense irregular connective tissue is composed mostly of fibrocytes and macrophages. White blood cells and adipose cells are typically not present in dense, irregular connective tissue.

Figure 3-7 is a photomicrograph of thin skin. Deep to the stratified squamous epithelium (see Stratified Squamous Epithelium section in Chapter 2, pp. 20–23) will be found *dense, irregular connective tissue* that comprises the bulk of the dermis of the skin. Collagen fibers dominate within this type of tissue, but reticular and elastic fibers may be present in varying amounts. The collagen fibers interlace considerably, forming a tough, latticelike network of fibers that may continue into adjacent tissues.

Dense Regular Connective Tissue

Tendons, aponeuroses, and ligaments are the most common examples of structures composed of dense regular connective tissue. Connective tissue fibers are arranged in a parallel fashion within this tissue, thereby giving the structures significant tensile strength.

Tendon

The histological identification of tendons and elastic (yellow) ligaments is quite difficult, but with adequate practice and side-by-side comparisons it can be readily accomplished.

Figures 3-8 and 3-9 are longitudinal H & E sections of a tendon. Tendons demonstrate collagen fibers that are closely packed and parallel and that appear quite homogenous. Because of the fixation process, these fibers are frequently wavy in appearance. In addition, because such preparations often vary in thickness within the field of vision, staining intensity may vary considerably, with the preparation being lighter in some sections of the field of vision and darker in others. Such fixation and staining artifacts are quite common in this tissue and are evident in Figure 3-8.

Fibrocytes are the only cell type found within this form of connective tissue and are to be found lying between the fiber bundles. These cells are typically elongated in appearance and have prominent nuclei. The location of the fibrocytes, their shape, and the manner in which they appear to be "regularly arranged" between the fiber bundles is a major histological feature of tendons.

Elastic Ligament

Collagenous ligaments are quite similar to tendons in composition and histological appearance because they are composed of a mixture of collagen and elastic fibers. Other ligaments, such as elastic ligaments (yellow ligaments), may be composed entirely of elastic fibers. As with tendons, fixation and staining artifacts may be quite common in ligament preparations.

Figures 3-10 and 3-11 are photomicrographs of an elastic ligament. Note that the elastic fibers appear as structureless, homogenous threads that branch and anastomose frequently. The fibers are dense and approximately parallel.

Fibrocytes are the only cell type present within ligaments; they do not appear as elongated as the fibrocytes seen in tendons (Figures 3-8 and 3-9). Ligaments (particularly elastic ligaments) may be distinguished from tendons in that fibrocytes nuclei are not found between the fiber bundles. Rather, the fibrocyte nuclei are found among the individual fibers. Because of this, the arrangement of the fibrocytes in an elastic ligament appears more random in comparison with that seen in tendons.

Commonly Misidentified Tissues

Dense Regular Connective Tissue: Tendon and Elastic Ligaments

Tendons and ligaments are examples of dense regular connective tissue. Both are characterized by the close packing of connective tissue fibers, and both occur in the form of sheets, bands, and cordlike structures. In addition, fibrocytes are the only cell type found in both of these structures. These similarities, as well as common changes that occur during fixation, make the differentiation between tendon and ligament quite difficult.

Tendon (Review **Figures 3-8** and **3-9** in Tendon section, pp. 50–52)

1. Fibrocytes are relatively few in number.

2. Fibrocytes are found between the bundles.

3. Fibrocytes tend to be elongated in shape.

Ligament (Elastic Type) (Review **Figures 3-10** and **3-11** in Elastic Ligament section, pp. 50, 53, 54)

1. Fibrocytes appear more numerous than in tendons.

2. Fibrocytes are found among the bundles of fibers.

3. Fibrocytes tend to be less elongated.

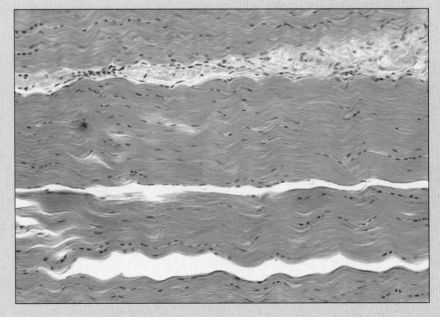

Figure 3-7 (100×): Dense irregular connective tissue (dermis of the skin).

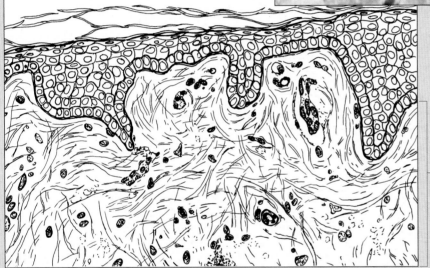

Dense irregular connective tissue

Figure 3-8 (35×): Tendon (dense regular connective tissue).

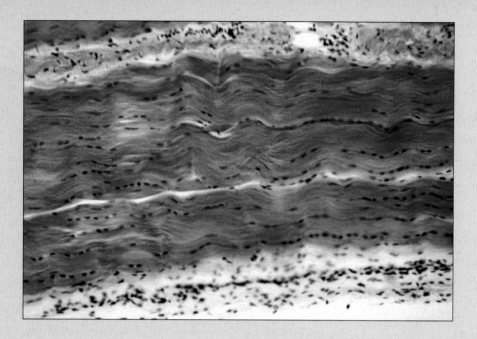

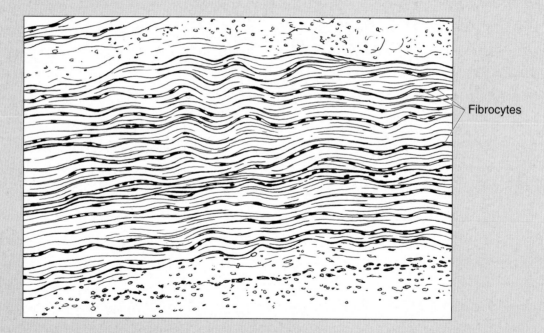

Fibrocytes

Figure 3-9 (50×): Tendon (dense regular connective tissue).

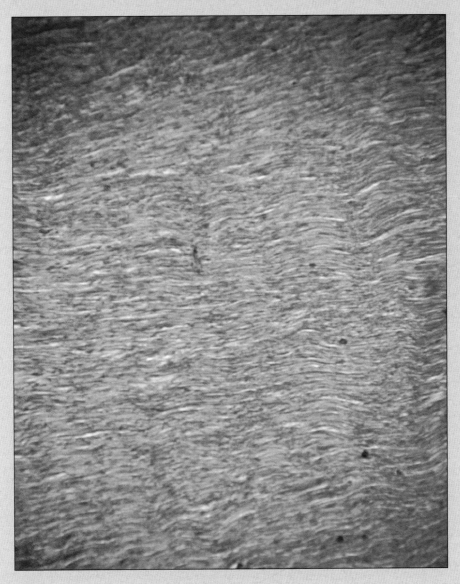

Figure 3-10 (25×): Ligament (elastic type) (dense regular connective tissue).

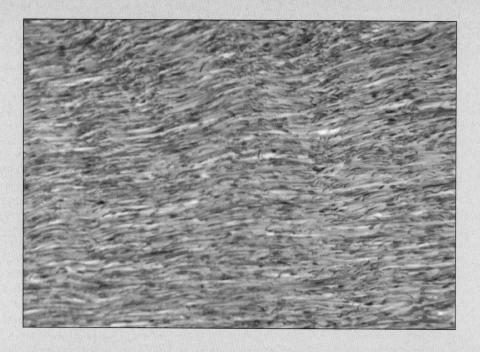

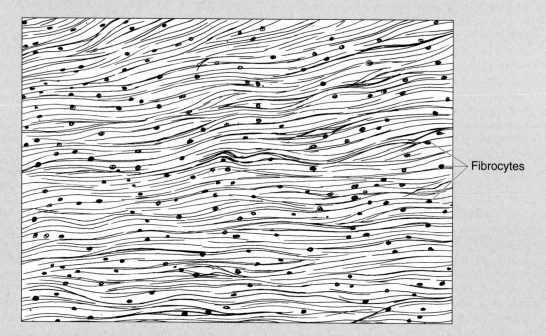

Fibrocytes

Figure 3-11 (50×): Ligament (elastic type) (dense regular connective tissue).

Chapter 4

SPECIALIZED CONNECTIVE TISSUE

Chapter Objectives

This chapter will enable you to:

1. Differentiate among the three types of cartilage

2. Differentiate among the different cell types normally found in cartilage

3. Identify the components of the perichondrium

Characteristics of Cartilage

Like other forms of connective tissue, cartilage is composed of cells and an extracellular matrix of fibers and ground substance. However, cartilage differs from previously studied forms of connective tissue in several ways:

- Mature cartilage is avascular.

- Cartilage is not penetrated by any element of the nervous system.

- The cells of cartilage, termed *chondrocytes*, are interspersed within the ground substance of cartilage and are to be found trapped within small, cavity-like spaces termed *lacunae*.

- The ground substance of cartilage has a gel-like consistency, which gives the tissue an elastic firmness capable of withstanding large amounts of pressure and shearing forces.

Subcategories of Cartilage

Cartilage is subdivided into three categories: hyaline, elastic, and fibrous cartilage (fibrocartilage). These different types of cartilage are distinguished by the appearance and components of the ground substance and fibers and by the presence or absence of an outer fibrous layer of connective tissue termed the *perichondrium*.

- Hyaline cartilage is the most common of the three forms of cartilage. It will be found in numerous locations, including the articulating surfaces of synovial joints, the cartilage model of developing long bones, the epiphyseal growth plates of long bones, and as supporting structures within the respiratory tree.

- Fibrous cartilage is typically found in areas of considerable stress. Because of the arrangement of fibers within the extracellular matrix, fibrous cartilage is better able to withstand compressive and shearing forces than the other forms of cartilage. Fibrous cartilage will be found within the pubic symphysis, annulus fibrosus of intervertebral discs, articular discs of the temporomandibular and sternoclavicular joints, and the menisci within the knee joint. It is also found in the areas of transition between cartilage and bone and forming the linkage between tendons and bones.

- Elastic cartilage is the least common of the three forms. It is found within the auricle of the external ear, the auditory tube of the middle ear, and the epiglottis.

Hyaline Cartilage

Hyaline Cartilage (Trachea)

As you examine these photomicrographs, it is important to keep in mind that *hyaline cartilage should be the reference by which you judge all other cartilages. If you know the histological characteristics of hyaline cartilage, you can use them to compare and contrast all other unknown cartilage specimens and thereby arrive at a correct tissue identification.*

As mentioned earlier, the best way to begin an initial examination of a new preparation or the identification of an unknown tissue is to start on scanning power (Figure 4-1) and then slowly progress to medium power (Figure 4-2) and high-dry (Figure 4-3) objectives.

The trachea is held open by C-shaped pieces of hyaline cartilage. As you begin your examination of Figure 4-1 you will see hyaline cartilage surrounded by adipose tissue and skeletal muscle. You will note that the hyaline cartilage is surrounded by dense regular connective tissue termed the *perichondrium.*

Continued examination shows that the interior of the cartilage is composed of cells, termed *chondrocytes,* which are trapped within spaces called *lacunae.* The prominence of these lacunae within the collagen is due to the shrinkage of the chondrocytes during fixation—a *fixation artifact* commonly seen in hyaline cartilage preparations. This fixation artifact creates an artificial space between the chondrocyte and the walls of its lacuna.

Hyaline cartilage stained with hematoxylin and eosin (H & E) demonstrates an unevenly stained matrix between the chondrocytes and their lacunae (Figure 4-2). The matrix between lacunae is typically homogeneous and lightly basophilic, although that may vary from preparation to preparation. The area immediately surrounding each lacuna or groups of lacunae typically stains more intensely and is termed the *territorial matrix.* The lighter-staining matrix between cell groups is termed the *interterritorial matrix.*

Because the fibers of hyaline cartilage are at or below the resolution of the light microscope and therefore are not visible with H & E, the matrix of hyaline cartilage appears "glassy," a major histological feature of hyaline cartilage.

Now turn your attention to Figures 4-2 and 4-3, and begin your examination at the periphery of the cartilage. Hyaline cartilage is surrounded by a connective tissue structure termed the *perichondrium.* The perichondrium serves an important role during growth and repair of hyaline cartilage.

The perichondrium is composed of two layers. The outer layer, termed the *fibrous perichondrium,* is composed of dense, irregular connective tissue. The spindle-shaped cells found within this layer of the perichondrium are *fibrocytes.* The inner layer of the perichondrium is termed the *chondrogenic layer.* The cells found within this layer are rounder and larger than the fibrocytes found within the outer, fibrous layer. These cells are termed *chondroblasts* and are responsible for the secretion of the ground matrix of the hyaline cartilage. Chondroblasts secrete large amounts of collagenous fibers and the hyaluronic acid and chondroitin of the matrix. Because the refractive indices for the chondroitin sulfate and collagen at the periphery of the cartilage matrix are quite similar, the collagenous fibers are poorly visible.

Now continue your examination of Figures 4-2 and 4-3 by moving deeper within the cartilage. As the chondroblasts continue to secrete the collagen, hyaluronic acid, and chondroitin sulfate, the cells become confined to restricted areas termed *lacunae.* When a chondroblast becomes trapped within a lacuna, it differentiates, becomes known as a *chondrocyte,* and is responsible for maintaining the cartilaginous matrix. Immediately surrounding the lacunae of hyaline cartilage you will note the *capsule.*

In mature cartilage, a chondrocyte will completely fill the lacuna. However, these photomicrographs present you with a very common fixation artifact—namely, the shrinkage of the chondrocyte such that it no longer fills the lacuna.

Note that some lacunae are occupied by two or more chondrocytes. Such a structure is termed a *chondrocyte aggregate* (isogenous group). Cartilage grows by two quite different processes—appositional growth and interstitial growth. These chondrocyte aggregates are the result of interstitial growth.

Toward the periphery of the cartilage there is a gradual transition from true cartilage to the surrounding perichondrium. This gives evidence of the second kind of cartilage growth, which is known as *appositional growth.* In young cartilage, interstitial growth predominates; in older cartilage, appositional growth predominates.

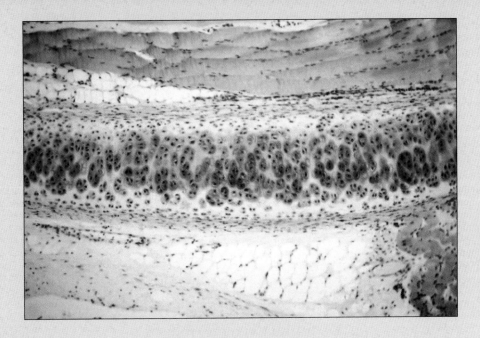

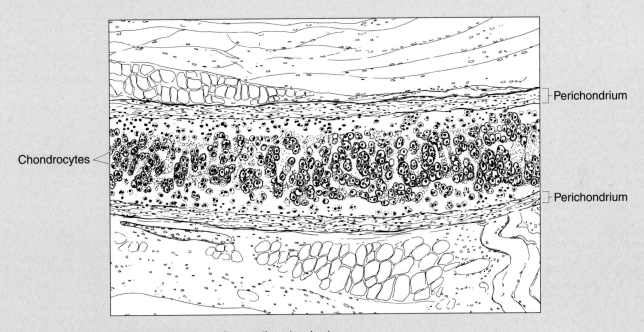

Figure 4-1 (50×): Hyaline cartilage (trachea).

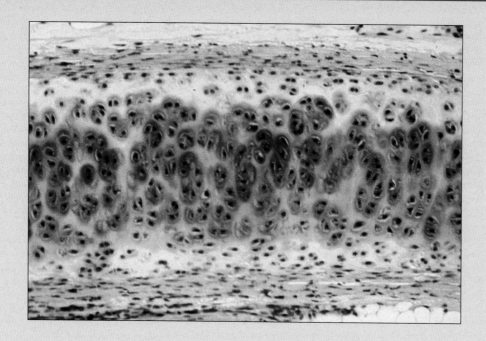

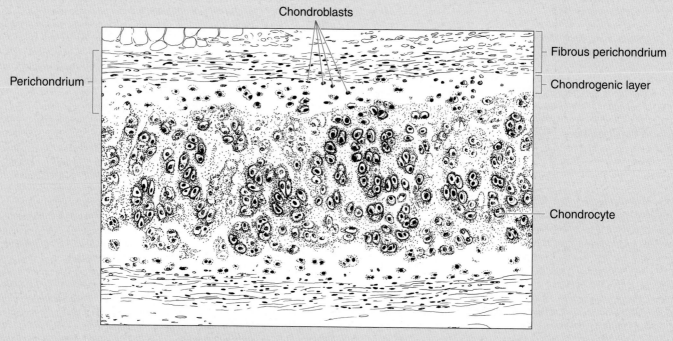

Figure 4-2 (100×): Hyaline cartilage (trachea).

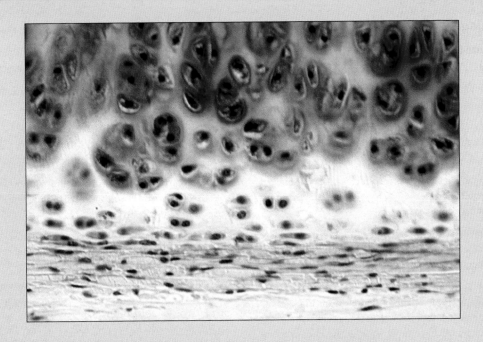

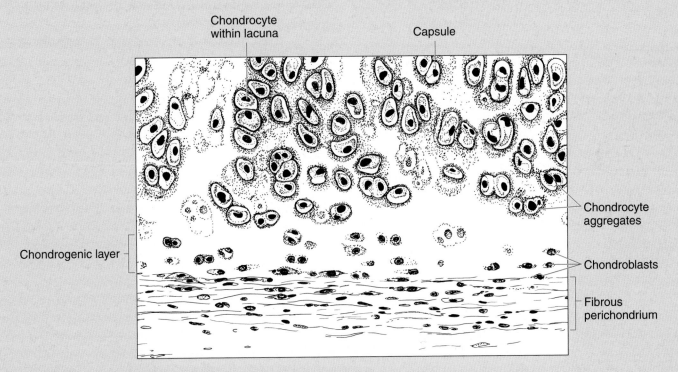

Figure 4-3 (200×): Hyaline cartilage (trachea).

Elastic Cartilage

Elastic Cartilage (Auricle of the Ear) (Elastin Stain)

As you examine Figures 4-4 and 4-5, you will note several similarities between hyaline cartilage (see Figures 4-1 to 4-3) and elastic cartilage:

- Elastic cartilage, like hyaline cartilage, possesses a perichondrium.

- As in hyaline cartilage, the perichondrium surrounding elastic cartilage is composed of an outer fibrous layer and an inner chondrogenic layer.

- The fibrous layer of the perichondrium in elastic cartilage is dense, regular connective tissue. The dominant cell type within this layer is the fibrocyte, just as in hyaline cartilage.

- The chondrogenic layer of the perichondrium in elastic cartilage possesses chondroblasts, with histological characteristics identical to those seen in the chondrogenic layer of hyaline cartilage.

Continued examination of elastic cartilage will show you that the *chondrocytes* of elastic cartilage are similar to the chondrocytes of hyaline cartilage (see Figures 4-1 to 4-3) in many ways:

- Chondrocytes of elastic cartilage are contained within *lacunae.*

- As in hyaline cartilage, a *capsule* surrounds the periphery of the lacunae.

- Chondrocytes of elastic cartilage may be found singly or in *chondrocyte aggregates* of two to four cells.

Closer examination of the chondrocytes within the lacunae of elastic cartilage will show several important differences when compared with those found within hyaline cartilage (see Figures 4-1 to 4-3):

- The chondrocytes of elastic cartilage are usually flatter.

- Chondrocytes of elastic cartilage have a more pointed shape.

Finally, the most obvious difference between hyaline and elastic cartilage is the appearance of the ground substance of elastic cartilage. In elastic cartilage, the ground substance is permeated with frequently branching elastic fibers. These elastic fibers form a network that often is so dense that it obscures the ground substance from view. This characteristic, when combined with the shape of chondrocytes within elastic cartilage, makes the identification of elastic cartilage quite easy.

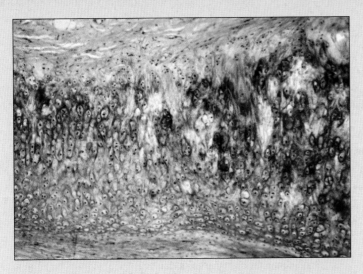

Figure 4-4 (50×): Elastic cartilage (auricle of the ear) (elastin stain).

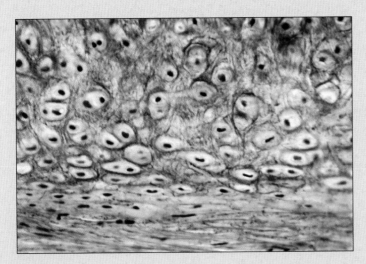

Figure 4-5 (200×): Elastic cartilage (auricle of the ear) (elastin stain).

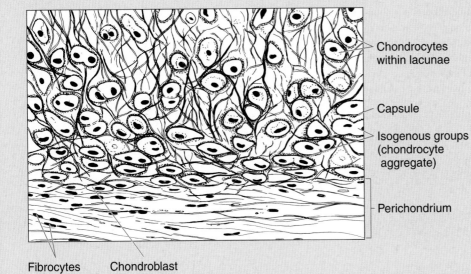

Chondrocytes
within lacunae

Capsule

Isogenous groups
(chondrocyte
aggregate)

Perichondrium

Fibrocytes   Chondroblast

Fibrous Cartilage

Fibrous Cartilage (Pubic Symphysis)

As you compare fibrous cartilage (fibrocartilage) in Figure 4-6 to hyaline cartilage (see Figures 4-1 to 4-3) and elastic cartilage (see Figures 4-4 and 4-5), you will note several striking similarities and differences.

As with hyaline and elastic cartilage, in fibrous cartilage the *chondrocytes* are contained within *lacunae*. However, there are several notable differences in the lacunae of fibrous cartilage:

- First, although *capsules* are present, they are not as prominent in fibrous cartilage as they are in hyaline or elastic cartilage.

- Note that the *lacunae are more regularly arranged (often being arranged into rows)* in fibrous cartilage, compared with the more random arrangement seen in hyaline and elastic cartilage.

Continued examination reveals that the interterritorial matrix of fibrous cartilage is not as homogenous as that of hyaline cartilage. Indeed, you will see collagen fibers within the cartilage matrix. You will also note that the collagenous fibers are more or less regularly arranged. These characteristics are important histological features of fibrous cartilage.

Fibrous cartilage is found in locations of high stress. The regular arrangement of the fibers within the matrix tends to follow the compression and shear forces to which the particular piece of fibrous cartilage is subjected.

Although elastic cartilage (see Figures 4-4 and 4-5) also presents a nonhomogenous matrix, fibrous cartilage differs from elastic cartilage in at least two ways:

- First, the fibers visible within the matrix of fibrous cartilage are more regularly arranged than those seen within the matrix of elastic cartilage.

- Second, the collagen fibers dominant within fibrous cartilage matrix stain acidophilic, whereas elastic fibers dominant within the matrix of elastic cartilage stain black in color.

Finally, fibrous cartilage often serves as a continuum between cartilage and bone or tendon and bone. In such instances, you will note that fibrous cartilage often lacks a peripheral perichondrium. This histological characteristic will vary, however, from location to location. The fibrous cartilage associated with many articulations, including the tibiofemoral menisci, glenoid labrum, and the discs of the acromioclavicular joint may possess a perichondrium, as evidenced by the capacity for limited cartilage repair at these joints.

Commonly Misidentified Tissues

Hyaline Cartilage and Fibrous Cartilage

If you do not closely examine sections of hyaline cartilage and fibrous cartilage, it is easy to confuse these two tissue types. Confusion may also arise if the section you are examining does not contain a perichondrium because of the plane of section. Therefore it is important to keep these characteristics in mind:

Hyaline Cartilage (Review **Figures 4-1** to **4-3** in section on Hyaline Cartilage [Trachea])

1. Matrix homogeneous in appearance

2. Possesses a perichondrium

3. Lacunae randomly arranged

4. Capsule readily seen

5. Chondrocyte aggregates commonly observed in tissue

Fibrous Cartilage (Review **Figure 4-6** in section on Fibrous cartilage [Pubic Symphysis])

1. Collagenous fibers are readily seen in matrix.

2. Perichondrium is lacking.

3. Lacunae are more widely spaced and more regularly arranged.

4. Capsules are seldom seen.

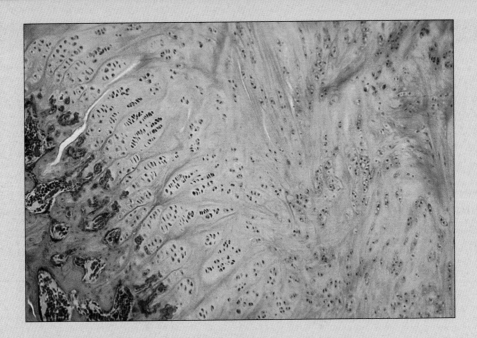

Chondrocytes within lacunae

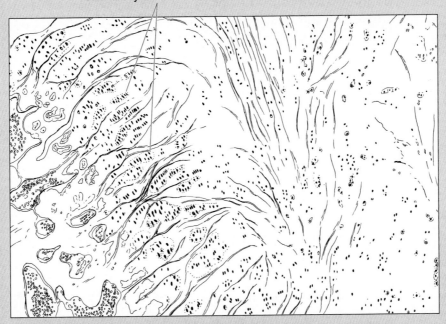

Figure 4-6 (100×): Fibrous cartilage (pubic symphysis).

Logic Tree

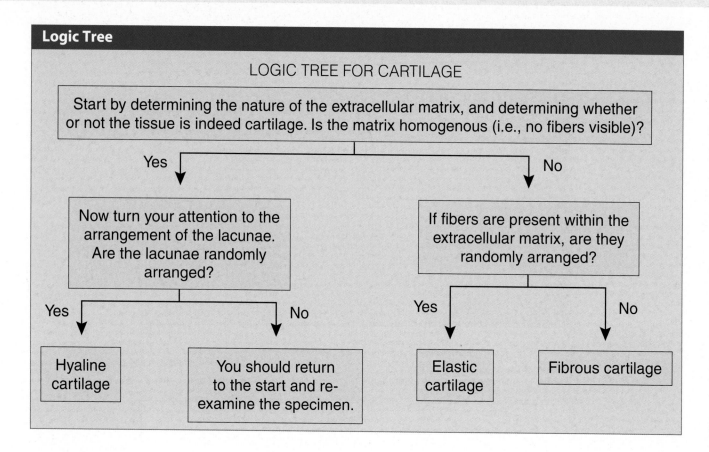

LOGIC TREE FOR CARTILAGE

Start by determining the nature of the extracellular matrix, and determining whether or not the tissue is indeed cartilage. Is the matrix homogenous (i.e., no fibers visible)?

Yes — Now turn your attention to the arrangement of the lacunae. Are the lacunae randomly arranged?

Yes → Hyaline cartilage

No → You should return to the start and re-examine the specimen.

No — If fibers are present within the extracellular matrix, are they randomly arranged?

Yes → Elastic cartilage

No → Fibrous cartilage

SPECIALIZED CONNECTIVE TISSUE: BONE

Histological Similarities Between Bone and Cartilage

Bone and cartilage are different forms of connective tissue. As a result, as you progress through this chapter you will note a considerable number of histological similarities and differences between cartilage (particularly hyaline cartilage; see section on hyaline cartilage in Chapter 4) and bone. Some similarities are:

- Bone and cartilage both consist of cells embedded within a matrix of organic and inorganic materials.

- Cartilage and bone both have cells trapped within lacunae.

- Bone and cartilage, particularly hyaline and elastic cartilage, both possess a bilayered connective tissue covering.

Histological Differences Between Bone and Cartilage

You will see several histological differences between bone and cartilage:

- Bone has a greater ratio of cells to amorphous ground substance.

- The bilayered connective tissue covering bone is termed the *periosteum*.

- The matrix in bone is composed primarily of hydroxyapatite crystals, hence the need for blood vessels and cell-to-cell contact for nourishment and the elimination of wastes. Therefore mature bone is highly vascular.

Cells of Bone

Four different cell types will be found within mature bone: osteoprogenitor cells, osteoblasts, osteocytes, and osteoclasts.

Osteoprogenitor cells are located on the external and internal surfaces of bones. Surrounding the external surface of all bones is a layer of connective tissue termed the *periosteum*. In addition, lining the marrow cavity of long bones is another, considerably thinner layer of connective tissue, the *endosteum*. The periosteum is divided into two layers: an outer fibrous layer and an inner osteogenic layer. Osteoprogenitor cells are found in the innermost layer of the periosteum, where they are called *periosteal cells*. They are also found in the endosteum, where they are termed *endosteal cells*. Endosteal cells are also found in the connective tissue lining the central (Haversian) and penetrating (Volkmann's) canals of mature bone. Osteoprogenitor cells typically differentiate into osteoblasts, although they may also differentiate into adipocytes or fibroblasts.

Histologically, osteoprogenitor cells have the following characteristics:

- Thin, attenuated, flattened shape

- Lightly staining, elongated or ovoid-shaped nuclei

- Variably staining cytoplasm, ranging from lightly acidophilic to lightly basophilic

The second cell type found in mature bone is the *osteoblast*. The primary function of osteoblasts is the synthesis and secretion of the collagenous fibers and ground substance of bone. In addition, osteoblasts participate in the ossification process by the secretion of matrix vesicles containing alkaline phosphatase.

Osteoblasts are found immediately deep to the periosteum and endosteum of mature bone. These cells have the following histological characteristics:

- Large cells that are rounded or polygonal in shape

- A single, eccentrically placed nucleus, typically found in the portion of the cell farthest from the developing bone

- Deeply basophilic-staining cytoplasm, nucleus, and nucleolus resulting from active protein synthesis

The third cell type found in mature bone is the *osteocyte*. An osteocyte is a mature cell trapped within a lacuna; it is responsible for maintaining the bony matrix. Osteocytes have the following histological characteristics:

- They are found within a lacuna within the bony matrix.

- The nucleus stains lightly basophilic, whereas the cytoplasm does not stain or will stain lightly acidophilic because of the reduced synthetic activity of the cell.

- They are slightly smaller in size than an osteoblast.

- They have thin, cytoplasmic processes that extend into the canaliculi of the bony matrix.

Osteoclasts are the fourth cell type of mature bone. These are large cells that are responsible for synthesis of the enzymes essential for the reabsorption of bone matrix during the remodeling of bone. Osteoclasts are found in two locations in mature bone: (1) associated with the inner portion of the endosteum, and (2) located within a depression termed a *resorption bay* (osteoclast crypt or Howship's lacuna).

Osteoclasts exhibit the following histological characteristics:

- They are large, multinucleate cells.

- The cytoplasm will usually stain acidophilic but may vary in staining intensity, depending on the synthetic activity of the cell.

Adult bone may be divided into two subcategories: compact bone (also termed *lamellar, dense,* or *cortical* bone) and trabecular *(spongy* or *cancellous)* bone. Compact bone is typically limited to the cortex or outer layer of adult bones; it is quite strong and heavy.

Trabecular bone, in contrast, generally lies within the interior of the bone, including the expanded epiphyseal ends of long bones. Trabecular bone provides strength with minimal weight.

The histology of bone depends on the age and level of development of the specimen. Developing, immature, and mature bones exhibit considerable histological differences. To understand the histology of mature, adult bone, it is essential to develop an understanding of the development, or osteogenesis, of bone.

Bone Development

Membranous Bone Development

Bone develops by two mechanisms: membranous (also termed *intramembranous* development) and endochondral (*intracartilaginous* development). Membranous ossification occurs in the formation of bones such as the clavicle, mandible, and the flat bones of the face and skull.

Membranous bone development occurs within vascularized embryonic mesenchyme. Briefly, mesenchymal cells in close proximity to the newly arrived blood vessels differentiate into osteoblasts and establish centers of ossification. Osteoblasts will secrete the organic matrix first, followed by the inorganic matrix, thereby forming bony spicules or trabeculae. Osteoblasts become increasingly farther apart as additional matrix is synthesized. As they become separated, osteoblasts develop thin, cyto-

plasmic processes, which enable intercellular communication via gap junctions. As the osteoblasts become trapped within lacuna, they differentiate and are termed *osteocytes*.

Initially, the newly formed bone is trabecular in nature. Further development may result in the formation of compact bone with its corresponding osteons (Haversian systems).

Membranous Bone Development (Fetal Pig)

As discussed earlier, during membranous (intramembranous) bone development embryonic mesenchyme develops a rich vascular network, and the embryonic mesenchymal cells develop long, tapering processes that enable the cells to maintain contact with one another. The spaces between the cells soon become occupied with bundles of collagenous fibers. Mesenchymal cells then differentiate into osteoprogenitor cells, which ultimately differentiate into osteoblasts, cells that are responsible for membranous bone development.

Figure 5-1 demonstrates slender eosinophilic (acidophilic) *bone spicules* developing within embryonic *mesenchyme*. Closer examination of a series of these spicules in **Figures 5-2** and **5-3** will illustrate the processes that occur during membrane bone development.

Figures 5-2 and **5-3** demonstrate small spicules of bone within the embryonic mesenchymal tissue. The periphery of the bony spicules is surrounded by basophilic *osteoblasts*. In the center of the spicules, note the *osteocytes* trapped within *lacunae*.

As you examine **Figure 5-3**, you will note a narrow region directly deep to the osteoblasts that stains differently when compared with the rest of the bony matrix. The developing bone in this narrow region is termed *osteoid*. Osteoid is the organic matrix of the developing bone that has been laid down by the osteoblasts but has not yet undergone ossification.

Osteoclasts are giant, multinucleate cells located within a *resorption bay* (also termed an *osteoclast crypt* or *Howship's lacuna*), a depression on the periphery of the bony matrix. Osteoclasts are often incorrectly identified because several osteocytes may be stacked on top of one another, thereby resembling an osteoclast. Although not foolproof, following is a trick to locating an osteoclast on your laboratory slides and preventing a misidentification of this cell type:

- Scan the specimen on low or medium power and look for a cell that is significantly larger than any other in the field. (Note the cell indicated on **Figure 5-2**.)

- On locating such a cell, switch to high-dry objective and determine how many nuclei are in the cell in question. (Now note the corresponding cell on **Figure 5-3**.)

- If the cell appears to be multinucleate, you must determine whether or not it actually is an osteoclast. The easiest way to do this is to slowly alter the fine focus and see whether all (or most) of the nuclei come into and out of focus simultaneously. If they do, you have located an osteoclast; if not, you have probably located several osteoblasts stacked on top of each other, as indicated by the nuclei being within different planes of focus.

- Because some osteoclasts have nuclei in multiple planes of focus, this method of identifying multinucleate cells is not foolproof.

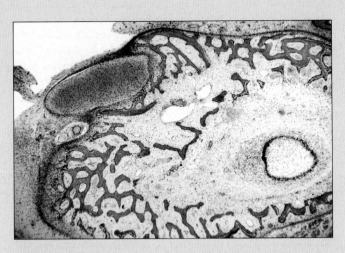

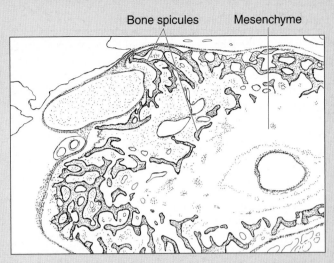

Figure 5-1 (25×): Membranous bone development (fetal pig).

Bone spicules   Mesenchyme

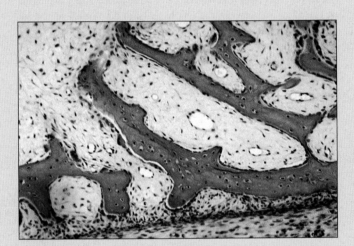

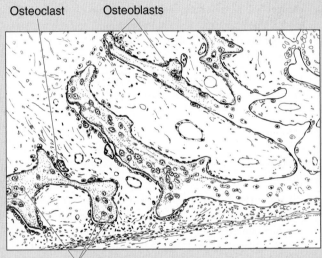

Osteoclast   Osteoblasts

Osteocytes within lacunae

Figure 5-2 (50×): Membranous bone development (fetal pig).

Osteocytes within lacunae   Osteoclast

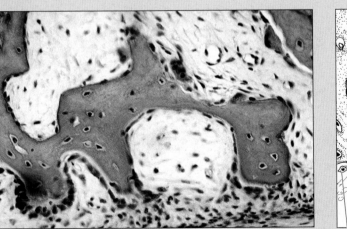

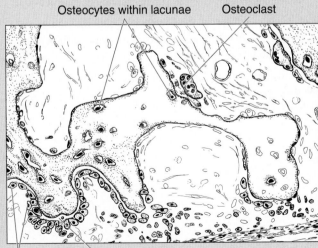

Osteoblasts   Osteoid

Figure 5-3 (100×): Membranous bone development (fetal pig).

Endochondral Bone Development

The bones of the limbs and other bones that bear weight, such as the vertebral column, develop by endochondral (intracartilaginous) ossification. This type of ossification starts with the formation of a cartilage model, which is then replaced with bone by the process outlined below.

The first step is the formation of a hyaline cartilage model of the long bone. All subsequent ossification will occur within this model. Endochondral ossification occurs initially within the diaphysis of the bone in an area termed the *primary ossification center*. The following steps will occur at the primary ossification center:

- The perichondrium surrounding the cartilage model differentiates into a periosteum as osteoprogenitor cells form within the periosteum. These cells will differentiate into osteoblasts, and osteoblasts will secrete a bony collar around the diaphysis of the hyaline cartilage model.

- Subsequent to the formation of the bony collar, histological changes will be observed within the interior of the cartilage model. The chondrocytes will hypertrophy, and the matrix surrounding them will calcify. Subsequently, the chondrocytes within the calcified matrix die.

- The newly developed periosteum increases in vascularity, and these newly formed capillaries invade the cartilage model of the bone.

- Osteoprogenitor cells from the periosteum will migrate into the interior of the calcified cartilage model, following the capillaries from the periosteum. These cells will then differentiate into osteoblasts.

- Osteoblasts will secrete bone within the center of the cartilage model. Initially, this newly formed bone is secreted on and around the calcified cartilage matrix within the center of the cartilage model. Therefore the first bone formed by this process will surround a core of cartilage. Because of the different staining properties of cartilage and bone, these trabeculae will have a spotty or mottled appearance. This spotty appearance is seen only within the center of the cartilage model of the newly forming bone; the bone laid down immediately deep to the periosteum is compact bone.

- Subsequently, the calcified cartilage within the center of the cartilage model will be removed, and newly synthesized bone will take its place.

As ossification progresses within the diaphysis of the bone, the process will begin to repeat at the expanded epiphyseal ends of the bone. These newly formed ossification centers at the epiphyseal ends are termed *secondary ossification centers*. As ossification progresses within the secondary ossification centers, the hyaline cartilage that remains between the diaphysis and the epiphysis is termed the *epiphyseal plate*. This epiphyseal plate will ultimately separate the epiphyseal and diaphyseal portions of the developing bones and is responsible for increasing the length of the developing bone.

Endochondral Ossification at the Epiphyseal Region (Fetal Metatarsal Bone)

Figure 5-4 shows a fetal metatarsal bone at the junction between the epiphyseal and diaphyseal regions. Note that the *epiphyseal region* on the right is composed of *hyaline cartilage*. A secondary ossification center has not yet developed in the epiphyseal end, but note the invasion of the hyaline cartilage by several vascular elements. The *primary ossification center* is located within the *diaphysis* of the developing bone.

Figure 5-5 is a higher magnification of the same distal (epiphyseal) end of a fetal metatarsal bone. Bone formation is occurring at the junction between the epiphyseal and diaphyseal regions of the bony model, which is seen at the left in this photomicrograph.

The hyaline cartilage within the epiphyseal end of a developing long bone will demonstrate a characteristic zonation as the epiphyseal plate begins to form. Beginning at the distal end of the bone and progressing toward the junction with the diaphysis you will see the following zones:

- *Resting Zone (zone of resting or reserve cartilage)*. This zone is composed of typical hyaline cartilage.

- *Proliferation Zone*. Cells within this zone are undergoing cellular division and are aligning themselves into distinct rows parallel to the longitudinal axis of the developing bone.

- *Hypertrophic Zone (zone of maturation)*. This zone contains chondrocytes that have enlarged considerably. In addition, chondrocytes within this zone accumulate glycogen, which will be dissolved during the fixation process.

- *Calcification Zone*. The cells within this narrow zone have begun to degenerate, and the matrix surrounding them is beginning to calcify.

Figure 5-6 shows bony spicules within the diaphysis of the developing bone. Note the *osteoblasts* located on the periphery of the developing bone. *Osteocytes* are seen trapped within *lacunae* of the spicule.

Epiphyseal region

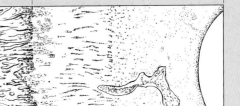

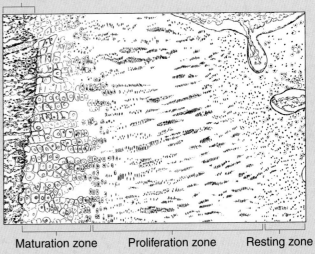

Primary ossification center

Figure 5-4 (40×): Endochondral ossification at the epiphyseal plate (fetal metatarsal bone).

Calcification zone

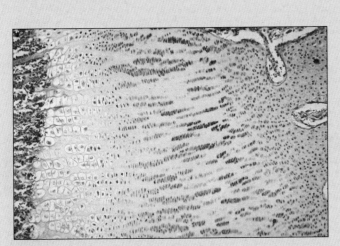

Maturation zone　　Proliferation zone　　Resting zone

Figure 5-5 (25×): Endochondral ossification at the epiphyseal plate (fetal metatarsal bone).

Osteoid

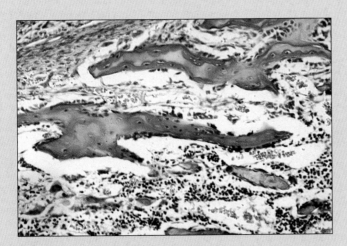

Osteocytes within lacunae　　Osteoblasts

Figure 5-6 (50×): Bony spicules within the diaphysis of the developing bone (intracartilaginous development) (fetal metatarsal bone).

Mature Bone

Mature bone may be in the form of compact or trabecular (cancellous) bone. Trabecular bone is composed of slender, interlacing bony trabeculae. Marrow is located within the spaces between the trabeculae. Both types of mature bone are organized into layers, called *lamellae*. Trabecular bone presents parallel lamellae, whereas compact bone presents circular lamellae.

Compact Bone—Cross Section—Ground Bone

Figure 5-7 is a cross section of ground, compact bone obtained from the diaphysis of a long bone. Because of this style of tissue preparation, the inorganic matrix is maintained, and the organic components (blood vessels, cells, and unmineralized matrix) are absent.

Compact bone is organized into a lamellar arrangement termed *osteons* (Haversian systems). Osteons consist of concentric, circumferentially arranged lamellae of osteocytes within *lacunae* and a *central* (Haversian) *canal*. Also visible in this figure is a *perforating* (Volkmann's) *canal* connecting two central canals.

The remodeling of bone continues throughout the life of an individual. Changes in an individual's level of physical activity will produce variations in stress at tendon and ligament attachment sites that contribute to bone remodeling. As bone is remodeled, new bone is deposited, and other areas of older bone are reabsorbed. *Interstitial lamellae* are the result of this remodeling process. These are fragments of osteons of older bone that persist following the reabsorption of older bone and the deposition of newer bone during the remodeling process.

Figure 5-8 is an oil-immersion photomicrograph of a cross section of ground, compact bone. This figure demonstrates *lacunae* and their interconnecting *canaliculi*.

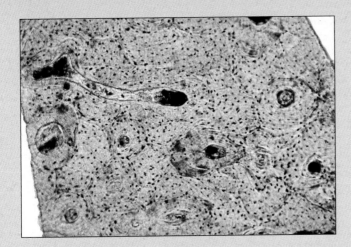

Figure 5-7 (25×): Compact bone (cross section)—ground bone.

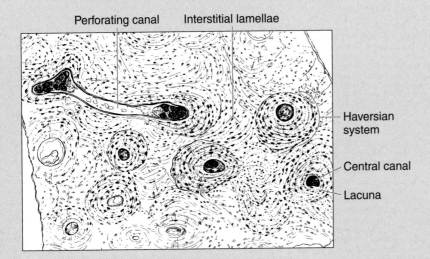

Perforating canal   Interstitial lamellae

Haversian system

Central canal

Lacuna

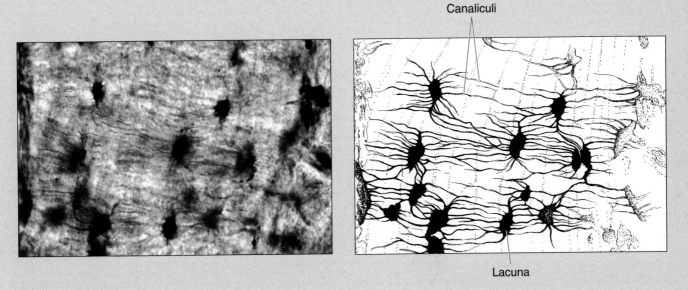

Canaliculi

Lacuna

Figure 5-8 (250×): Compact bone (cross section)—ground bone.

Periosteum

Figure 5-9 is a cross section of a decalcified, compact bone. At the periphery of this section you will note the *periosteum*. Because of the thickness of the specimen, note how the photomicrograph makes the transition from being in focus to out of focus as you scan the specimen from left to right. This is yet another example of specimen artifact, attributable either to the plane of section or the mounting of the specimen on the slide.

The periosteum is composed of two layers: an outer *fibrous layer* and an inner *osteogenic layer*. The fibrous layer is composed of dense connective tissue. The nuclei of *fibrocytes* found within this layer are visible.

The inner layer of the periosteum is termed the *osteogenic layer*. Within this layer are osteoprogenitor cells and *osteoblasts*.

Osteoprogenitor cells (not visible in this photomicrograph) are flattened, resting cells with the ability to differentiate into *osteoblasts* that are visible in the inner portion of the periosteum.

What accounts for the histological differences seen among Figures 5-9 (decalcified bone), 5-7, and 5-8 (ground bone)?

Trabecular Bone

Figure 5-10 is taken from the epiphysis of a long bone. The *trabeculae* (bony spicules) throughout this figure are immature and still undergoing osteogenesis, as evidenced by the variations in the staining characteristics. Compare the histological appearances of trabecular (cancellous) and compact bone (see Figures 5-7 and 5-8). What would be a major difference between these two forms of mature bone?

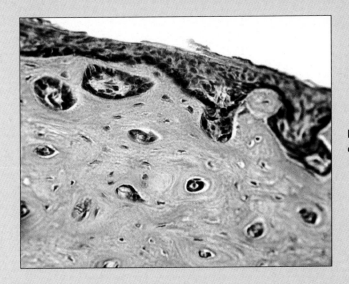

Figure 5-9 (100×): Cross section of decalcified, compact bone demonstrating periosteum.

Osteoblast within osteogenic layer
Fibrocyte within fibrous layer

Periosteum

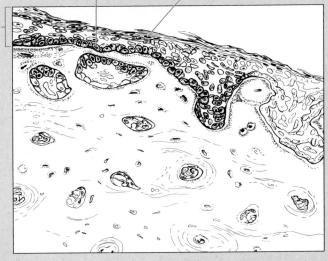

Trabeculae

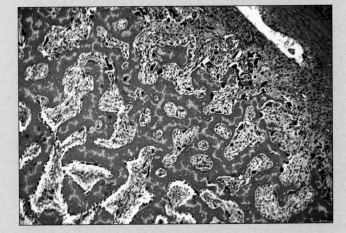

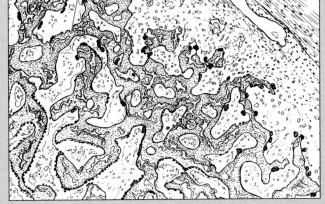

Figure 5-10 (50×): Trabecular bone.

Chapter 6

MUSCLE TISSUE

Chapter Objectives

This chapter will enable you to:

1. Differentiate among the varying types of muscle tissue when viewed in cross and longitudinal sections.

2. Differentiate among endomysium, perimysium, and epimysium and be able to explain the various components found within these connective tissue investments.

3. Identify myosatellite cells and explain their function.

4. Identify intercalated discs in cardiac muscle and explain their function.

Types of Muscle

Human muscle tissue is classified into the following categories: skeletal striated muscle and noncardiac visceral striated muscle,* smooth muscle, and cardiac striated muscle. These categories are based on the location, function, and structure of the tissue.

Skeletal striated muscle (skeletal muscle) is the most abundant of the muscle types in the human body. It is responsible for appendicular and axial skeletal movements. In addition to moving skeletal structures, skeletal muscles are also responsible for moving the eyes, tongue, deep fascia, and skin of the face. Skeletal muscle cells possess "stripes" or striations. These striations (A band and I band) are the result of differences in light passage and absorption in the tissue. Skeletal muscle is also termed *voluntary* muscle in that contractions can be initiated via the "voluntary" or somatic nervous system.

Cardiac muscle is limited to the heart and exhibits a banding pattern quite similar to that of skeletal muscle. Cardiac muscle is commonly called a *functional syncytium* in that excitation of one cardiac muscle cell will quickly cause the excitation of all adjacent cells via the intercalated discs found between the cells.

Smooth muscle is the only type that does not possess striations. Smooth muscle is typically found within the hollow visceral organs and blood vessels of the body and is functionally subdivided into "single unit" or "multi-unit" smooth muscle, depending on how easily action potentials may spread from one cell to another.

Skeletal Muscle

Skeletal muscle fibers demonstrate the following histological characteristics:

- Cells are long and cylindrically shaped.

- Cells are multinucleate.

- Nuclei are peripherally located.

- When viewed in longitudinal section, skeletal muscle cells demonstrate a regularly arranged banding pattern.

As you examine the following photomicrographs, it is important to keep in mind that skeletal muscle should be the reference by which you judge all other muscular tissue. If you know the histological characteristics of skeletal muscle (in both cross and longitudinal sections), you can then use these characteristics to identify all other unknown muscle specimens.

---

*As per the *Terminologia Histologica* (TH, 2008): "The following classification acknowledges the presence of nonskeletal, noncardiac striated muscle, such as esophageal striated muscle and external anal and urethral sphincters."

Skeletal Muscle—Cross Section

Figure 6-1 is a cross-sectional view of skeletal muscle. *Because skeletal muscle cells are cylindrical in shape, you will see very little size variation between the individual myofibers, a major histological feature of this tissue.* Although this cross section does not demonstrate the multinucleate nature of skeletal muscle fibers, it clearly demonstrates that the *nuclei are peripherally located, another major histological feature of skeletal muscle when viewed in cross section.*

Skeletal muscle has a rather complex connective tissue investment. The external surface of the entire muscle is covered with connective tissue, termed *epimysium*, which is not visible in this section. The epimysium then extends into the interior of the muscle as *perimysium*, which divides the skeletal muscle into *fascicles*. The *endomysium* is found surrounding each individual skeletal muscle cell, external to the basal lamina.

Figure 6-2 is a higher magnification of Figure 6-1 and demonstrates the *perimysium*, *endomysium*, and accompanying slender *fibrocytes*.

As you center your attention on the individual *myofibers*, you will see the *peripherally located nuclei*. In addition, you can distinguish *myosatellite* (satellite) *cells*. Myosatellite cells are stem cells that may divide and form additional myofibers following muscle injury. Myosatellite cells are found beneath the basal lamina of skeletal muscle cells and external to the sarcolemma (muscle cell membrane). They may be distinguished from fibrocytes by their more slender nuclei.

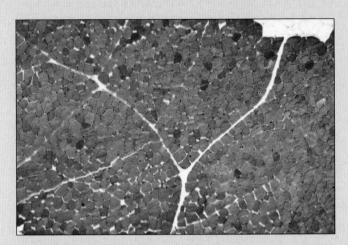

Figure 6-1 (25×): Skeletal muscle (cross section).

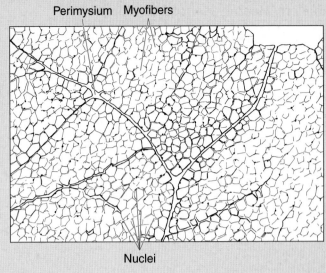

Figure 6-2 (100×): Skeletal muscle (cross section).

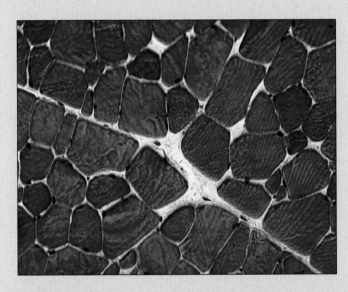

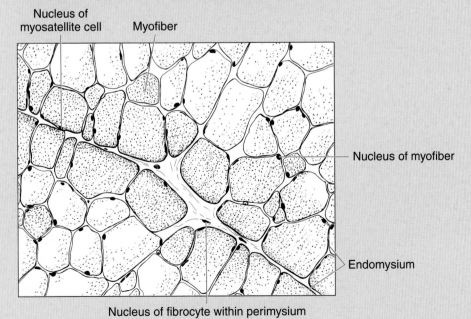

Skeletal Muscle—Longitudinal Section

Figures 6-3 and 6-4 demonstrate skeletal muscle in longitudinal section. *The banding pattern is clearly evident, as are the peripheral nuclei. Note how the banding pattern in skeletal muscle is "in register"(lined up) from one cell to another. This is a major histological feature of skeletal muscle when viewed in longitudinal section.*

Nuclei of *fibrocytes* located within the perimysium are also evident in **Figure 6-3.**

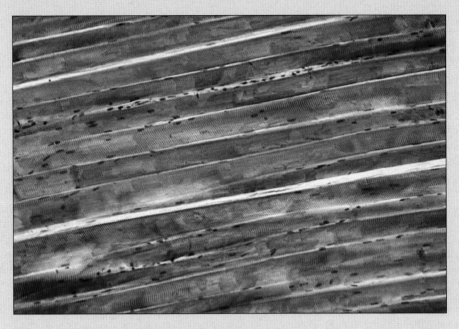

Figure 6-3 (50×): Skeletal muscle (longitudinal section).

Nuclei of myofibers

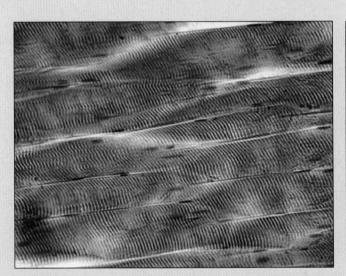

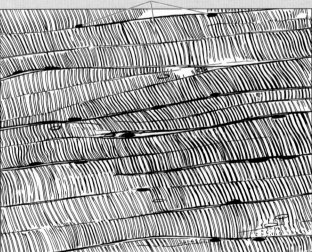

Figure 6-4 (100×): Skeletal muscle (longitudinal section).

Cardiac Muscle

Cardiac muscle, like skeletal muscle, is striated; however, that is where the histological similarities end. As you examine the following photomicrographs of cardiac muscle, keep in mind the following histological differences between skeletal and cardiac muscle:

- Cardiac muscle cells are considerably smaller than skeletal muscle fibers. The exception to this rule is Purkinje fibers, which will be studied in Chapter 8, the Cardiovascular System.

- Cardiac muscle cells branch frequently and therefore demonstrate a greater size variation when viewed in cross section.

- Cardiac muscle cells (except for Purkinje fibers) have a single, centrally located nucleus.

- Cardiac muscle cells possess specialized cell junctions called *intercalated discs*, and these are visible in longitudinal sections of cardiac muscle.

Figure 6-5 is a photomicrograph of cardiac muscle in longitudinal section. *Note that cardiac muscle usually has only one centrally located nucleus per cell.* In addition, note the sectioning artifacts at the periphery of this photomicrograph.

Figure 6-6 clearly demonstrates the *centrally located nuclei* and the *intercalated discs* found between adjacent cardiac muscle cells. Intercalated discs are specialized junctions that facilitate the spread of electrical impulses from one cardiac muscle cell to another. They also anchor cardiac muscle cells to one another, thereby allowing the spread of contraction forces.

Compare this figure to skeletal muscle in Figure 6-4. *Note:*

- *How cardiac muscle cells branch*

- *That the banding pattern of cardiac muscle is not as prominent as that of skeletal muscle*

- *That the banding pattern between individual cardiac muscle cells is not "in register," as was seen in skeletal muscle*

These three characteristics are all major histological features of cardiac muscle when viewed in longitudinal section.

You will also note, as you compare Figures 6-4 and 6-6, that cardiac muscle exhibits fibers running in several different directions. This results in the presence of cross, longitudinal, and oblique sections on the same slide because of the helical arrangement of cardiac muscle within the heart. *This can be a useful identification tool.*

Figure 6-7 is a photomicrograph of cardiac muscle in cross section. *This figure clearly demonstrates two major histological features of cardiac muscle when viewed in cross section:*

- *Note that the nuclei in cardiac muscle cells are centrally located.*

- *In addition, this tissue demonstrates an increased variation in cell size compared to skeletal muscle in cross section (see Figure 6-1). This increased size variation is due to the branching of cardiac myocytes.*

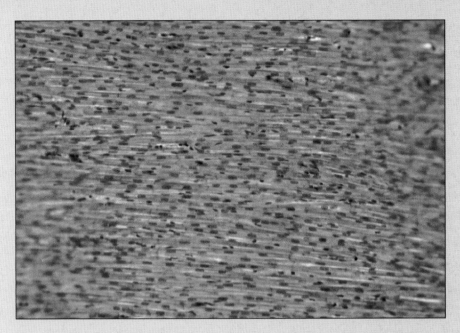

Figure 6-5 (50×): Cardiac muscle.

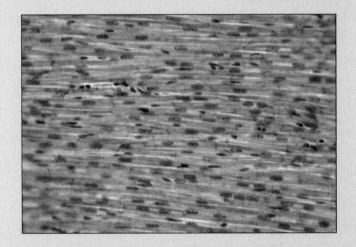

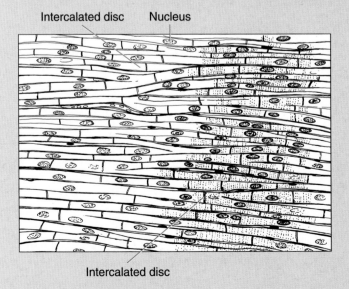

Intercalated disc   Nucleus

Intercalated disc

Figure 6-6 (100×): Cardiac muscle.

Smooth Muscle

As you examine the following photomicrographs of smooth muscle, you must compare smooth muscle to skeletal and cardiac muscle. As you make these comparisons, you will see the following similarities and differences:

- Smooth muscle, unlike cardiac and skeletal muscle, is not striated.

- Like cardiac muscle, smooth muscle has a single, centrally located nucleus.

- Smooth muscle cells, unlike skeletal and cardiac muscle, are fusiform in shape. Therefore they will demonstrate the greatest amount of size variation when viewed in cross section.

- Smooth muscle cells have long, football-shaped nuclei.

- The lateral borders of smooth muscle cells are quite difficult to see in hematoxylin and eosin preparations.

- Smooth muscle cells are much smaller than cardiac or skeletal muscle cells.

Figure 6-8 was taken from the smooth muscle found within the muscularis externa of the ileum of the small intestine. You can see smooth muscle in longitudinal section in this photomicrograph. (Note the sectioning artifacts at the periphery of this photomicrograph.)

When viewed in longitudinal section, smooth muscle cells are long and cigar shaped, appearing almost to interdigitate with each other. This reflects the overlapping of the individual smooth muscle cells.

Smooth muscle, when viewed in cross section, presents a considerable variation in cell and nucleus size. In addition, because of the shape of smooth muscle cells and the resulting plane of section, the number of cells possessing visible nuclei will also vary considerably throughout the field.

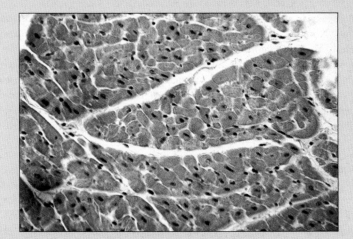

Figure 6-7 (100×): Cardiac muscle (cross section).

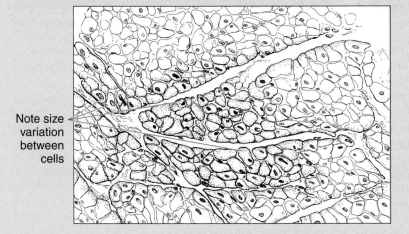

Note size
variation
between
cells

Nucleus within smooth muscle cell

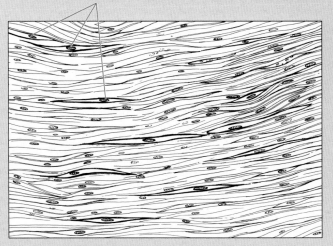

Figure 6-8 (50×): Smooth muscle from muscularis externa of
the ileum of the small intestine.

Figure 6-9 is a photomicrograph of smooth muscle in longitudinal and cross section taken at a higher magnification. Note the artifacts between the two layers of smooth muscle in this photomicrograph.

REFERENCES

Wareham AC, Whitmore I: A comparison of the mechanical properties of oesophageal striated muscle with skeletal muscles of the guinea pig, *Plflugers Arch* 395:312-317, 1983.

Whitmore I: The ultrastructure of oesophageal striated muscle in the guinea pig and marmoset, *Cell Tiss Res* 234:365-376, 1983.

Whitmore I: *2006 Terminologia histologica. International terms for human cytology and histology*, Philadelphia, Lippincott Williams & Wilkins.

Whitmore I, Gosling JA, Gilpin SA: A comparison between the physiological characteristics of urethral striated muscle in the guinea pig, *Pflugers Arch* 400:40-43, 1984.

Whitmore I, Notman JA: A quantitative investigation into some ultrastructural characteristics of guinea pig striated muscle, *Ann Anat* 153:233-240, 1987.

Commonly Misidentified Tissues

Skeletal, Smooth, and Cardiac Muscle

When viewing skeletal, smooth, and cardiac muscle it is important to keep in mind multiple aspects for comparison. The characteristics listed below are not the only factors that may be used for comparison but are the most obvious and will yield the best results with the least amount of effort.

Muscle and Section Type	Nucleus	Shape and Size Variation
Skeletal muscle (x.s.)	Multiple and peripheral	Rounded; 15-90 μM; minimal
Skeletal muscle (l.s.)	Multiple and peripheral	Rounded; 10-20 μM; minimal
Smooth muscle (x.s.)	Single and central	Circular; 7 μM; considerable
Smooth muscle (l.s.)	Single and central	Spindle shaped; considerable
Cardiac muscle (x.s.)	Single and central	Rounded; 10-20 μM; moderate
Cardiac muscle (l.s.)	Single and central	Branched; moderate

x.s, Cross section; *l.s.,* longitudinal section.

Note: The diameter of a red blood cell is 7 μM; this is a useful measurement tool for comparison when looking at these tissues.

Commonly Misidentified Tissues

Smooth Muscle, Tendon, and Ligament when Viewed in Longitudinal Section

Smooth Muscle/Longitudinal section (Review **Figures 6-8** and **6-9** in section on Smooth Muscle)

1. Fusiform or spindle-shaped cells with a single, centrally located, football-shaped nucleus

2. Nuclei aligned parallel with each other

3. Noticeable size variation in cells within preparation

4. Lack of "wavy" fibers in preparation

5. Relative homogeneous staining of preparation

6. Connective tissue investment surrounding smooth muscle cell bundles and individual cells

Dense Regular Connective Tissue: Tendon and Ligament/Longitudinal Section (Review **Figures 3-8** to **3-11** in section on Dense Regular Connective Tissue)

1. Long, thin, flattened nuclei within cells

2. Cells present distinctively smaller in size

3. Nuclei parallel with each other

4. "Wavy" appearance in preparation

5. Relative lack of homogeneous staining characteristics in preparation

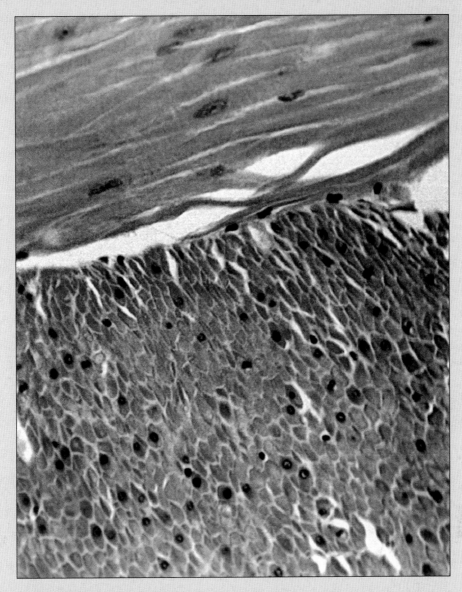

Figure 6-9 (100×): Smooth muscle from muscularis externa of the ileum of the small intestine (longitudinal and cross sections).

Logic Tree

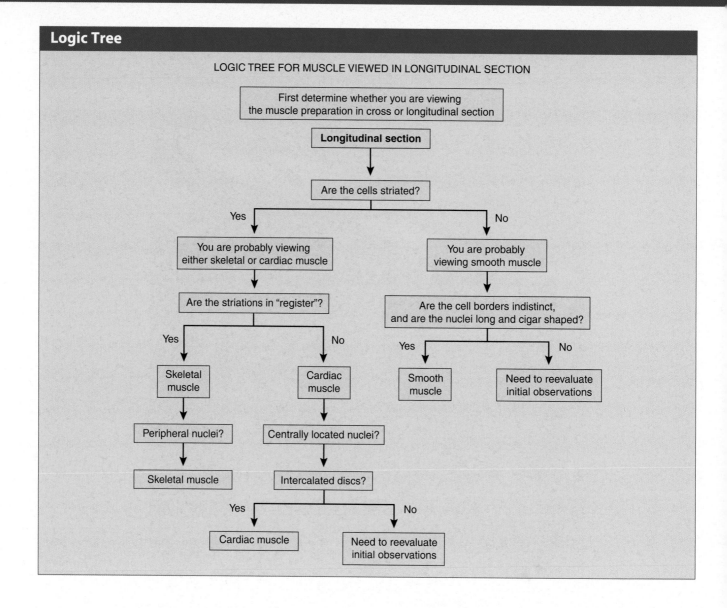

LOGIC TREE FOR MUSCLE VIEWED IN LONGITUDINAL SECTION

First determine whether you are viewing
the muscle preparation in cross or longitudinal section

Longitudinal section

Are the cells striated?

Yes — You are probably viewing either skeletal or cardiac muscle

No — You are probably viewing smooth muscle

Are the striations in "register"?

Yes — Skeletal muscle

No — Cardiac muscle

Are the cell borders indistinct, and are the nuclei long and cigar shaped?

Yes — Smooth muscle

No — Need to reevaluate initial observations

Peripheral nuclei? — Skeletal muscle

Centrally located nuclei?

Intercalated discs?

Yes — Cardiac muscle

No — Need to reevaluate initial observations

Logic Tree

LOGIC TREE FOR MUSCLE VIEWED IN CROSS SECTION

First determine whether you are viewing the muscle preparation in cross or longitudinal section.

Cross section

Are the nuclei peripherally or centrally located?

Peripherally located

Centrally located

You are probably viewing skeletal muscle

You are viewing either cardiac or smooth muscle

Look at the size variation of the individual myocytes.
Are the cells consistently the same size?

Look at the size variation of the individual myocytes.
Is the size variation considerable or moderate?

Yes

No

Considerable

Moderate

Skeletal muscle

Need to reevaluate initial observations

Smooth muscle

Cardiac muscle

NERVOUS TISSUE

The nervous system is composed of two cell types: neurons and glial supporting cells. Both of these cell types are found within the two subdivisions of the nervous system, the PNS and CNS. The CNS is composed of the brain and spinal cord, and the PNS consists of everything else.

The brain and spinal cord consist of white matter and gray matter. White matter is composed mostly of myelinated neuronal processes and supporting cells. Some unmyelinated processes may also be found within white matter. The gray matter is composed of neuronal somas, unmyelinated neuronal processes, and supporting cells.

While reading through this chapter you will notice that most of the specimens are represented twice: once stained with H & E and then with a heavy metal stain (silver). (See Appendix.) Study both types of specimens equally, because each of these stains will enable you to see different structures within each specimen. You should make constant mental notes as to which stain represents which structures most clearly. It is also important for you to keep in mind the gross anatomy of the central and peripheral nervous systems as you proceed through this chapter.

Central Nervous System

Spinal Cord

The spinal cord, when viewed in cross section, is composed of central gray matter and peripheral white matter. The gray matter resembles a butterfly in shape and may be subdivided into three pairs of horns: dorsal, lateral (found only between the first thoracic and second lumbar spinal levels), and ventral. Sensory neurons enter the spinal cord via the dorsal horn, whereas motor neurons originate within the lateral (autonomic nervous system, sympathetic branch) and anterior (somatic nervous system and autonomic nervous system, parasympathetic branch) horns.

Figure 7-1 is a line drawing of a cross section of the spinal cord. Use this line drawing to refresh your understanding of the gross anatomy of the spinal cord, paying particular attention to the following structures in this figure: *ventral horn, dorsal horn, white matter, gray matter, meninges, central canal, dorsal root ganglion, dorsal root of the spinal nerve,* and the *ventral root of the spinal nerve.*

Figure 7-2 is a photomicrograph of the anterior (ventral) horn of the spinal cord stained with H & E. The *neuronal cell bodies of the anterior horn cells* are quite large. They contain a single, large, centrally located *nucleus*. Several large *neuronal processes* exiting from the anterior horn cells are also evident in this section.

Many of the other nuclei found within the gray matter of the cord belong to *neural glial cells*. Their cytoplasm is not evident in these photomicrographs. The identification of the three types of glial cells within the CNS (microglia, astroglia, and oligodendroglia cells) requires the use of special stains and is not possible in these photomicrographs.

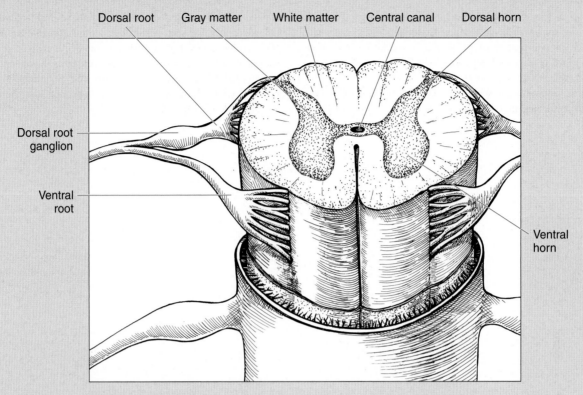

Dorsal root   Gray matter   White matter   Central canal   Dorsal horn

Dorsal root
ganglion

Ventral
root

Ventral
horn

Figure 7-1 Gross anatomy of a cross section of the spinal cord.

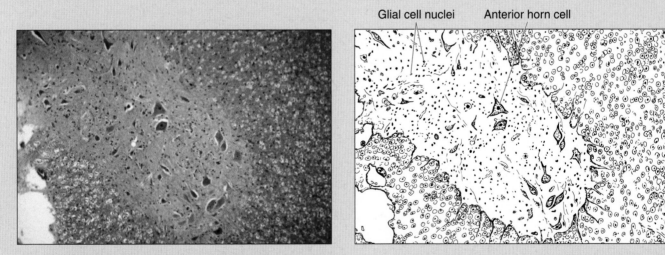

Glial cell nuclei   Anterior horn cell

Figure 7-2 (50×): Ventral (anterior) horn of the spinal cord.

Figure 7-3 is a photomicrograph of the anterior (ventral) horn of the spinal cord, viewed in cross section and stained with silver. As you compare this with Figure 7-2, what structures are stained more readily with silver than H & E? For which is the reverse true?

A cross section of the spinal cord at the junction of the *anterior horn* and peripheral *white matter* (see Figure 7-1) and stained with H & E is seen in Figure 7-4. Several large *neuronal cell bodies* may be seen within the central gray matter. Many of the smaller *nuclei* present within the white matter represent various *neuroglia*. The *axons* in true cross section appear as a dot surrounded by a white halo because the peripherally located myelin has dissolved during the fixation process and therefore is not available for staining.

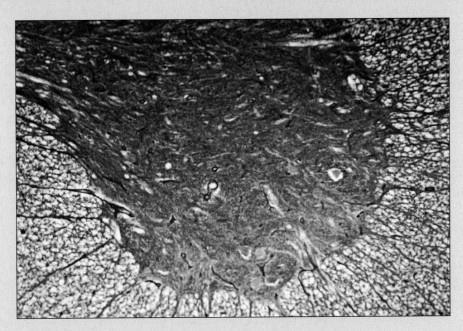

Figure 7-3 (50×): Ventral (anterior) horn of the spinal cord (silver stain).

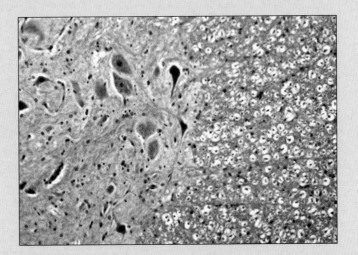

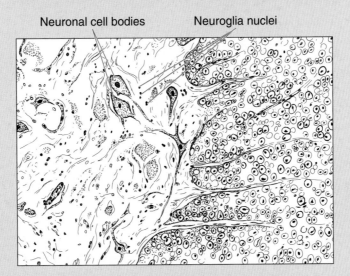

Neuronal cell bodies   Neuroglia nuclei

Figure 7-4 (100×): Cross section of the spinal cord at the junction of the anterior horn and peripheral white matter.

Figure 7-5 represents a silver stain of a cross section of the spinal cord at the junction of the *anterior horn* and peripheral *white matter* (see Figure 7-1). In the central gray matter you will note several large *neuronal cell bodies*. Central *nuclei* are visible in some of these cells. You will also see several *neuronal processes* exiting from the gray matter and entering the white matter.

Now compare the images seen in Figures 7-4 and 7-5. As you view the neurons and axons seen in Figure 7-4, what structures are clearly visible that are not seen in Figure 7-5? For which is the reverse true?

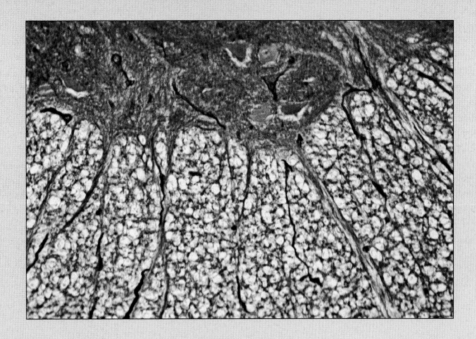

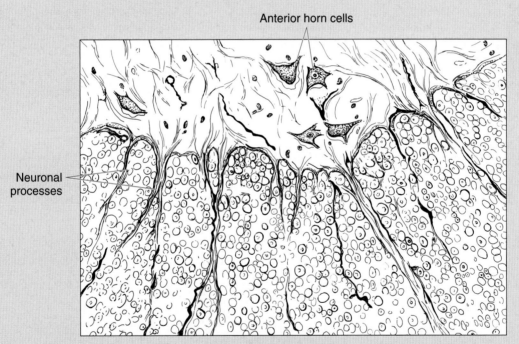

Figure 7-5 (100×): Cross section of the spinal cord at the junction of the anterior horn and peripheral white matter (silver stain).

Cerebellum

The surface of the cerebellum of the CNS is thrown into a large number of folds, termed *folia cerebelli*, which serve to increase the surface area of the cerebellum. The cerebellum is divided into a cortex of gray matter and a medullary center of white matter. The cerebellar cortex is divided into three layers: molecular, Purkinje, and granular. Each layer is named for the predominant cell type found within that layer.

Figures 7-6 and 7-7 are H & E photomicrographs of the cerebellar cortex. Note that the *cerebellar cortex* is composed of three layers: the outer *molecular layer* (sometimes termed the *plexiform layer*), which contains few cells and no myelinated fibers, an intermediate *Purkinje layer*, and the inner *granular layer*. Deep to the cortex is the histologically quite indistinct *white matter*.

In Figure 7-7 the border between the granular and molecular layers is the site of rather large neurons called *Purkinje cells, which are characteristic of the cerebellum*. Within the molecular layer you may be able to see basket cells. These neurons are quite small and demonstrate a small amount of cytoplasm around a centrally located nucleus.

In the granular layer, near its junction with the molecular layer, you may see occasional stellate neurons (also termed *Golgi cells*). These neurons are characterized by nuclei that are larger than those of the granule cells. Granule cells do not demonstrate the characteristic structure of neurons in that they possess dark nuclei, have no obvious nucleolus, and show no clearly stained cytoplasm. They are quite difficult to distinguish from glial cells.

Figure 7-8 is a silver stain of the junction between the *granular* and *molecular layers* of the cerebellum. Which neurons are visible within this photomicrograph?

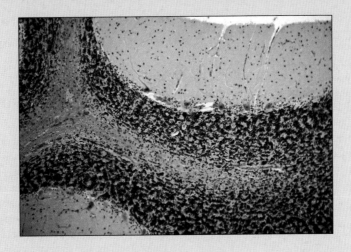

White matter

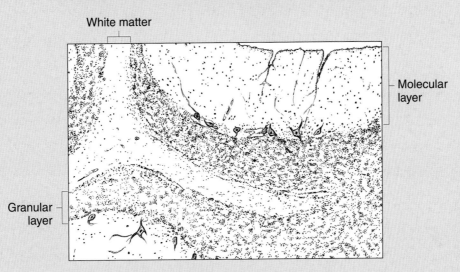

Molecular
layer

Granular
layer

Figure 7-6 (50×): Cerebellum.

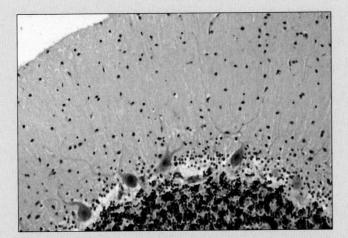

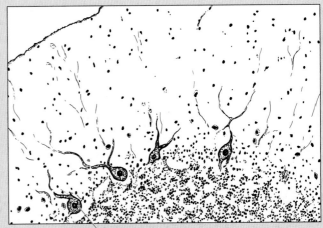

Figure 7-7 (200×): Cerebellum.

Purkinje cell

Cerebral Cortex

Ninety percent of the human cerebral cortex is neocortex (also termed *isocortex*), which is the phylogenetically newest and structurally most complex. The neocortex is composed of six layers that the beginning histology student will find difficult to distinguish. Each layer possesses several neuronal and glial cell types. These cells are not randomly arranged; one or more neurons dominate within each layer. Horizontal fibers associated with each layer also give a laminated appearance to the cortex.

The layers of the neocortex (from superficial to deep) and the neurons contained within them are as follows:

- Molecular layer: horizontal cells (also termed *horizontal cells of Cajal*)

- External granular layer: stellate (granule) cells

- External pyramidal layer: stellate cells and large pyramidal cells

- Internal granular layer: stellate cells

- Internal pyramidal layer: large and medium pyramidal cells

- Multiform layer: inverted pyramidal neurons (also termed *Martinotti cells*)

Figure 7-9 is a photomicrograph of the superficial layers of the cerebral cortex. You will note that *meninges* and associated *blood vessels* that normally cover the surface of the cerebral cortex are clearly visible. Within the molecular layer you will see the *horizontal neurons* (horizontal cells of Cajal). These relatively small cells are stellate or spindle shaped and their axons give rise to horizontally directed fibers. Deeper within the cerebral cortex are the large, triangular-shaped *pyramidal cells*.

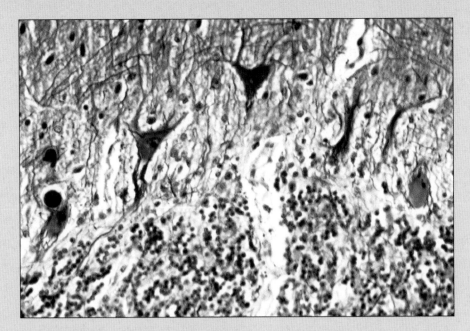

Figure 7-8 (200×): Cerebellum (silver stain).

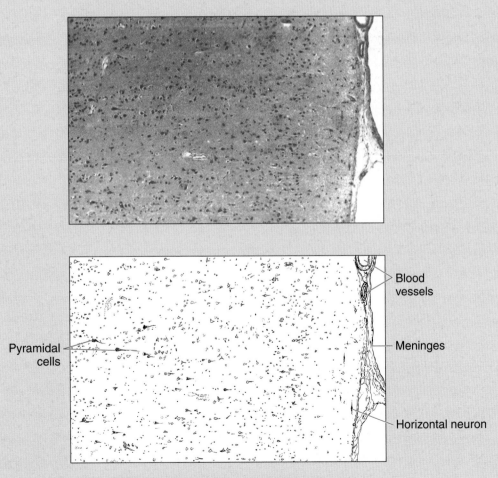

Figure 7-9 (50×): Cerebral cortex—superficial layers.

Blood vessels

Meninges

Pyramidal cells

Horizontal neuron

Peripheral Nervous System

Spinal Ganglion (Dorsal Root Ganglion)

Figures 7-10 and 7-11 demonstrate that the *neuronal somas* for sensory spinal nerves are located within the spinal (dorsal root) ganglia. Note the prominent, large, pale-staining *nucleus* and the smaller, darker-staining *nucleolus* within the soma. Also visible within these sections are horizontally aligned *myelinated axons*.

Surrounding the neuronal somas are *satellite cells*, a type of glial cell found with the peripheral nervous system.

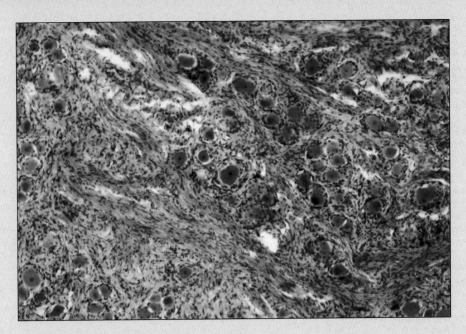

Figure 7-10 (50×): Dorsal root (spinal) ganglion.

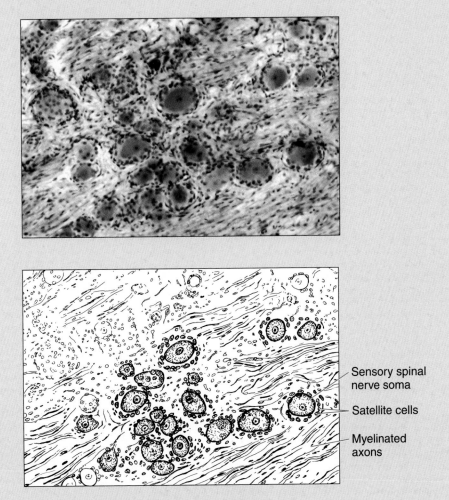

Sensory spinal
nerve soma

Satellite cells

Myelinated
axons

Figure 7-11 (100×): Dorsal root (spinal) ganglion.

Peripheral Nerve

Peripheral Nerve: Longitudinal Section

Figure 7-12 is a photomicrograph of a longitudinal section of peripheral nerve stained with H & E. At this magnification, several characteristics are apparent:

- Note the wavy appearance of the section. In addition, you will note several sections in which both longitudinal and cross sections are visible in this photomicrograph. Both of these are due to the recoil of the preparation during fixation and therefore are fixation artifacts.

- This longitudinal section is of a fasciculus of a peripheral nerve, thus the surrounding connective tissue is the *perineurium*.

- At this magnification, a longitudinal section of peripheral nerve may be easily confused with dense regular connective tissue (tendon) or smooth muscle.

Figure 7-13 is a photomicrograph of the same specimen taken at higher magnification. As you look at this specimen, note the following:

- The myelin sheath of these neurons has been dissolved away during the fixation process.

- A *centrally located axon* may be seen in some of the peripheral nerves.

- Several indentations may be seen in some of the myelin sheaths of the peripheral nerve. These indentations represent *myelin sheath gaps* (also termed *Nodes of Ranvier*).

- Numerous nuclei, which represent *Schwann cell* and *fibrocyte nuclei*, are evident in this figure.

Perineurium

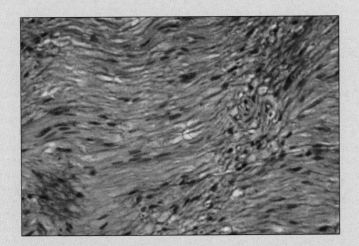

Figure 7-12 (100×): Peripheral nerve (longitudinal section).

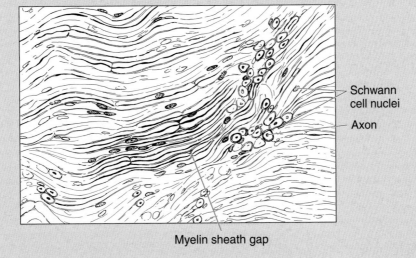

Schwann
cell nuclei

Axon

Myelin sheath gap

Figure 7-13 (200×): Peripheral nerve (longitudinal section).

Peripheral Nerve: Cross Section

Figures 7-14, 7-15, and 7-16 are photomicrographs of a large *peripheral nerve bundle* containing several smaller bundles within a connective tissue sheath. Each bundle, in turn, is composed of many large *peripheral axons*. Figures 7-14 and 7-15 were stained with H & E, and Figure 7-16 is a silver stain preparation.

As you progress from Figure 7-14 to 7-16, you will note the varying connective tissue investments: *epineurium, perineurium,* and *endoneurium.*

Figure 7-16 is a photomicrograph of peripheral nerve in cross section, stained with silver. Note the individual *axons*. The axons appear as a dot surrounded by a white halo because the myelin has been dissolved away during the fixation process.

As you compare Figures 7-14 through 7-16, what structures are more visible with silver stain than H & E? For which is the reverse true?

Several other questions are worth considering as you look at peripheral nerve in cross or longitudinal sections. In these photomicrographs, several nuclei are present. What cell types are represented by these nuclei? What cell type is definitely *not* represented by these nuclei here?

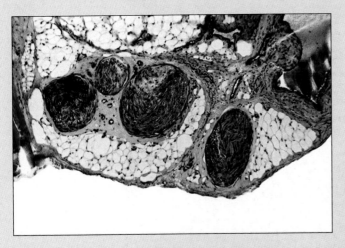 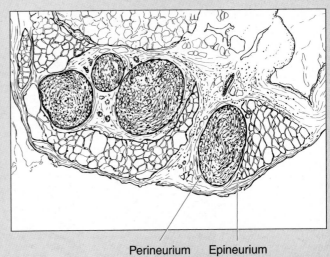

Perineurium   Epineurium

Figure 7-14 (50×): Peripheral nerve (cross section).

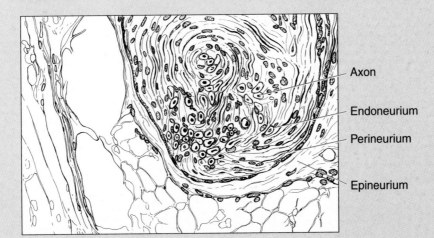

Axon

Endoneurium

Perineurium

Epineurium

Figure 7-15 (200×): Peripheral nerve (cross section).

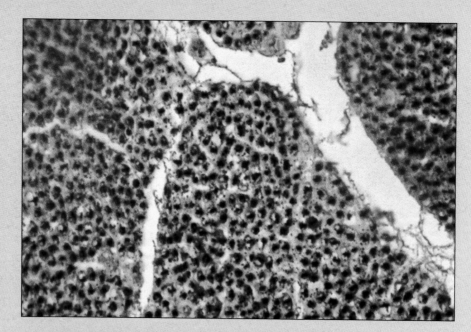

Figure 7-16 (200×): Peripheral nerve (cross section) (silver stain).

Peripheral Nerve: Autonomic Nervous System Ganglion

The gastrointestinal tract has rich autonomic nervous system innervation. Figures 7-17 and 7-18 demonstrate a *myenteric neural plexus* (also termed a *Myenteric Plexus of Auerbach*). This is a ganglion of the parasympathetic branch of the autonomic nervous system that is found between the *circular* and *longitudinal layers of smooth muscle* (see section on smooth muscle in Chapter 6 of the muscularis externa of the small intestine.) Individual *neuronal somas* with prominent *nuclei* are visible within this ganglion. Several blood vessels are also visible in these sections between the inner circular and outer longitudinal layers of smooth muscle.

Following are questions to consider for this structure:

- On the basis of what you know of anatomy, why is this a ganglion of the parasympathetic nervous system and not a ganglion of the sympathetic nervous system?

- The autonomic nervous system is a two-neuron system, composed of preganglionic and postganglionic neurons. Are the somas visible within this ganglion from preganglionic or postganglionic neurons? Why?

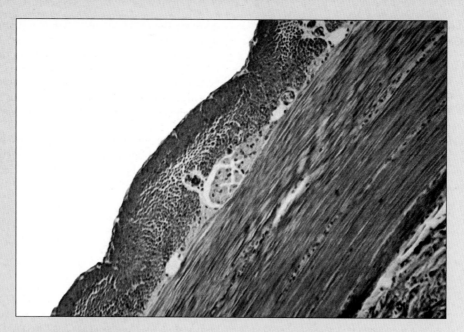

Figure 7-17 (100×): Myenteric neural plexus of the small intestine.

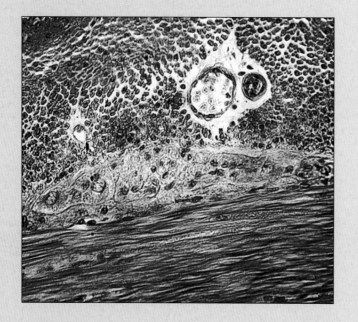

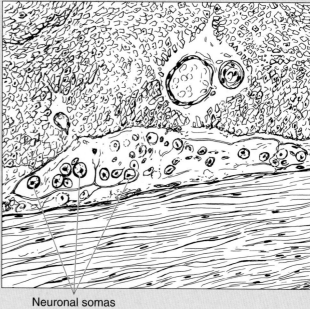

Neuronal somas

Figure 7-18 (200×): Myenteric neural plexus of the small intestine.

Commonly Misidentified Tissues

Peripheral Nerve, Dense Regular Connective Tissue (Tendon and Elastic Ligament)

Nervous tissue typically presents some identification problems. Peripheral nerve, smooth muscle, and dense regular connective tissue are often mistaken for each other and as a result are incorrectly identified. Therefore it is important for you to keep the following differences in mind when trying to differentiate between these different tissues:

Peripheral Nerve (Longitudinal Section) (Review **Figures 7-12** and **7-13** in section on Peripheral Nerve)

1. Presence of myelin sheath gaps (Nodes of Ranvier) under high-dry or oil-immersion objective

2. Generally "washed out" appearance of specimen

3. Axons surrounded by myelin sheath, which has been dissolved away during fixation process

4. Nuclei numerous and rounded (Schwann cells), or flat and dark (fibroblasts and fibrocytes)

5. Generally wavy appearance

6. Epineurium or perineurium present

Dense Regular Connective Tissue (Tendon and Elastic Ligament) (Longitudinal Section) (Review **Figures 3-8** to **3-11** in section on Dense Regular Connective Tissue in Chapter 3)

1. Absence of myelin sheath gaps (Nodes of Ranvier) under high-dry or oil-immersion objective

2. Fibers stained darkly; less wavy than peripheral nerve; more irregular in appearance

3. Nuclei more numerous and more evenly stained

4. Acidophilic collagen fiber bundles

5. Long, thin nuclei arranged in parallel

Peripheral Nerve and Smooth Muscle

Peripheral Nerve (Longitudinal Section) (Review **Figures 7-12** and **7-13** in section on Peripheral Nerve)

1. Presence of myelin sheath gaps (Nodes of Ranvier) under high-dry or oil-immersion objective

2. Generally "washed out" appearance of specimen

3. Nuclei numerous and rounded (Schwann cells), or flat and dark (fibroblasts and fibrocytes)

4. Generally wavy appearance

5. Blood vessels lacking (except in large nerves)

6. Epineurium or perineurium present

Smooth Muscle (Longitudinal Section) (Review **Figures 6-8** and **6-9** in section on Smooth Muscle in Chapter 6)

1. Absence of myelin sheath gaps (Nodes of Ranvier)

2. More uniform staining to general specimen

3. More uniformity in size, shape, and staining qualities of nuclei within specimen

Peripheral Nerve (Cross Section) (Review **Figures 7-14** and **7-15** in section on Cross Section of Peripheral Nerve)

1. Regular arrangement to connective tissue investment

2. Presence of "halos" around axons

3. Variation in staining qualities of nuclei within tissue

4. Large degree of uniformity in size of structures (axons) represented in cross section

5. Epineurium or perineurium present

Smooth Muscle (Cross Section) (Review **Figure 6-9** in section on Smooth Muscle in Chapter 6)

1. Decreased amount of connective tissue within specimen

2. Lack of myelin "halos"

3. Uniformity in staining qualities of nuclei within tissue

4. Considerable size variation of structures (myocytes) represented in cross section

CARDIOVASCULAR SYSTEM

The cardiovascular system consists of the heart and blood vessels. The histology of cardiac muscle has been discussed previously (Chapter 6). However, to place cardiac muscle within the context of the cardiovascular system, it is discussed again in this chapter.

Heart

Cardiac Muscle

Cardiac muscle is limited to the heart. The second form of striated muscle, it exhibits a banding pattern that is quite similar to that seen in skeletal muscle. Cardiac muscle is commonly called a *functional syncytium*, in that excitation of one cardiac muscle cell quickly causes the excitation of all adjacent cells. This is due to the specialized junctions, termed *intercalated discs*, which are found between cardiac muscle cells.

Cardiac muscle, like skeletal muscle, is striated; as a result, these two tissues are often misidentified. In Chapter 6 (see section on Cardiac Muscle) you were asked to keep in mind the following histological differences between skeletal and cardiac muscle:

- Cardiac muscle cells are considerably smaller than skeletal muscle fibers. The exception to this rule is Purkinje fibers.

- Cardiac muscle cells branch frequently and therefore demonstrate a greater size variation when viewed in cross section.

- Cardiac muscle cells (except for Purkinje fibers) have a single, centrally located nucleus.

- Cardiac muscle cells possess specialized cell junctions called *intercalated discs*, which are visible in longitudinal sections of cardiac muscle.

Figure 8-1 is a photomicrograph of cardiac muscle in longitudinal section. Note that cardiac muscle has only *one centrally located nucleus per cell*. Compare nucleus location and size variation demonstrated in this photomicrograph with that seen in comparable cross sections of skeletal muscle (see Figures 6-1 and 6-2).

Figure 8-2 clearly demonstrates the *single, centrally located nucleus* of cardiac muscle cells. *Intercalated discs,* seen between adjacent cardiac muscle cells, are specialized junctions that facilitate the spread of electrical impulses from one cardiac muscle cell to another. They also anchor adjacent cardiac muscle cells to one another, thereby allowing the spread of contractile forces from one cell to another within the heart.

Compare this figure to skeletal muscle in Figure 6-4. *Note the following characteristics of cardiac muscle; they will help you to differentiate between skeletal and cardiac muscle when viewed in longitudinal section:*

- *Note how cardiac muscle cells branch.*

- *Note that the banding pattern of cardiac muscle is not as prominent as that of skeletal muscle.*

- *Note that the banding pattern between individual cardiac muscle cells is not "in register," as was seen in skeletal muscle.*

These three characteristics are all major histological features of cardiac muscle when viewed in longitudinal section.

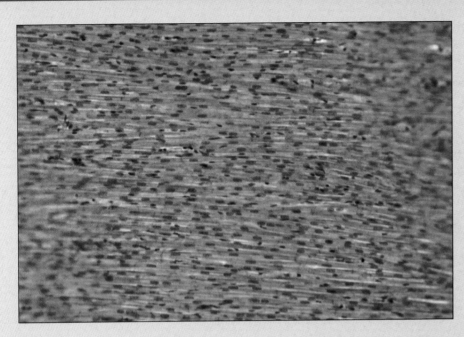

Figure 8-1 (100×): Cardiac muscle (longitudinal section).

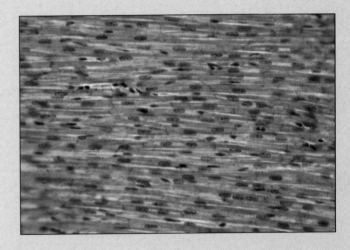

Figure 8-2 (200×): Cardiac muscle demonstrating intercalated discs (longitudinal section).

Intercalated disc   Nuclei

Intercalated disc

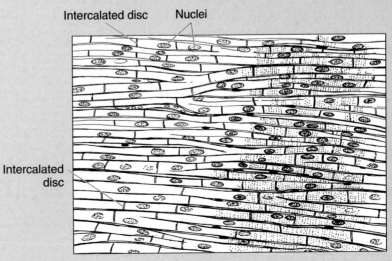

Figure 8-3 is a photomicrograph of cardiac muscle in cross section. This figure clearly demonstrates *two major histological features of cardiac muscle when viewed in cross section:*

- *Note that cardiac muscle has only one, centrally located nucleus per cell.*

- *In addition, this tissue demonstrates an increased variation in cell size compared with skeletal muscle viewed in cross section (see* Figure 6-1). *This increased size variation is due to the branching of the cardiac myocytes.*

Cardiac Muscle—Purkinje Fibers

Purkinje fibers are a part of the subendocardiac conducting network of the heart. Purkinje fibers are cardiac muscle cells specialized for high-velocity transmission of electrical impulses throughout the ventricle. Figure 8-4 demonstrates that Purkinje fibers:

- Usually occur in bundles

- Demonstrate a significantly increased muscle fiber diameter compared to other cardiac muscle cells

- Have an increased intracellular glycogen content, resulting in lighter staining properties

- Have a reduced number of myofibrils, and therefore a reduction in the banding pattern (when viewed in longitudinal section)

- Are multinucleate. The nuclei are more rounded and often found in groups of two or three within a single Purkinje fiber.

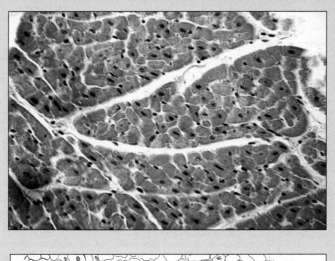

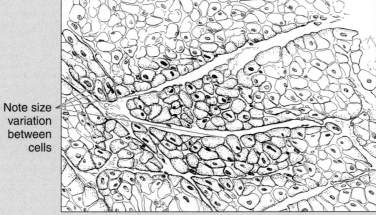

Note size
variation
between
cells

Figure 8-3 (200×): Cardiac muscle (cross section).

Purkinje fiber bundles

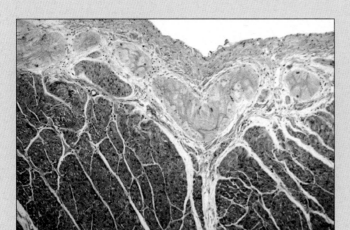

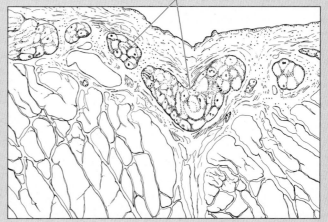

Figure 8-4 (50×): Cardiac muscle demonstrating Purkinje fibers.

Blood Vessels

All blood vessels within the cardiovascular system, with the exception of capillaries, follow the same histological organization. The walls of arteries, arterioles, veins, and venules all have three layers, or tunics.

- The innermost layer is the intima (or tunica intima), which consists of an endothelial tube of longitudinally arranged, simple, squamous epithelial cells termed *endothelial cells.*

  - A sheet of elastic tissue, termed the *internal elastic membrane (internal elastic lamina)*, forms the boundary between the intima and the second layer of the vessel, the media (or tunica media).

  - The thin, squamous endothelial cells are separated from the internal elastic membrane by a layer of loose connective tissue termed the *subendothelial connective tissue.* The subendothelial connective tissue contains a few fibrocytes, occasional smooth muscle cells, and thin collagen fibers.

- The media is composed of multiple concentric layers of circularly arranged, smooth muscle cells.

  - An external elastic membrane *(external elastic lamina)* serves as the boundary between the media and the outermost layer of the vessel, the adventitia (or tunica adventitia).

  - In larger vessels you may find small blood vessels, termed *vasa vasorum*, within the media. The vasa vasorum serve to nourish the vessel.

- The adventitia consists of fibrocytes, longitudinal bundles of collagen fibers, and a loose network of thin elastic fibers.

  - In larger vessels, vasa vasorum may also be found within the adventitia.

Arterial System

Elastic Arteries (Aorta)

Figure 8-5 is a cross section of a section of the aorta, an elastic artery, stained with hematoxylin and eosin.

The *intima* of an elastic artery is much thicker than its counterpart in a muscular artery, sometimes amounting to 20% of the total wall thickness. The intima of the aorta is composed of an *inner endothelial lining* that is continuous with the endothelial lining of the heart. The rounded nuclei of the endothelial cells may appear to project into the lumen of the vessel.

The external border of the intima is marked by an internal elastic membrane, which is not easily distinguished because of the large amount of elastin within the media of the vessel.

The *media* constitutes the bulk of the wall of an elastic artery and is composed of circularly arranged smooth muscle (see section on Smooth Muscle in Chapter 6) and a large number of fenestrated elastic membranes. These elastic membranes contain numerous openings termed *fenestrae*. The number of elastic laminae is believed to increase with age until approximately age 35.

At the outermost limit of the media is an external elastic membrane *(external elastic lamina)*, but this layer is usually indistinguishable in the aorta, again because of the large amount of elastin within the media.

The *adventitia* of an elastic artery is usually quite thin. It consists of irregular connective tissue with collagen and elastic fibers, some fibroblasts, and smooth muscle cells. *Vasa vasorum* are visible in this figure.

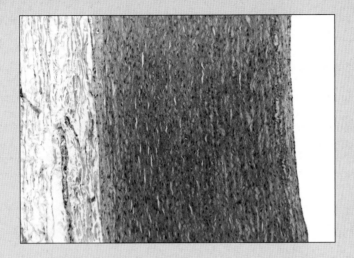

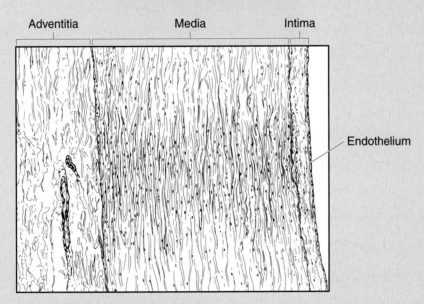

Figure 8-5 (50×): Aorta (elastic artery).

Muscular Arteries

Figure 8-6 is a photomicrograph of a muscular artery *(right)* and a vein *(left)*, and Figure 8-7 is a higher magnification of the wall of a muscular artery.

Note the conspicuous *intima* in the muscular artery. The external limit of the intima is marked by an *internal elastic membrane*, which is convoluted because of the contraction of the elastic membrane during the fixation process.

The *media* of a muscular artery is composed of many circumferentially arranged smooth muscle cells. The media ends abruptly with a well-defined but thinner *external elastic membrane*.

Beyond the media is the *adventitia*. The adventitia contains circumferentially arranged *fibrocytes* and collagen fibers arranged both circumferentially and longitudinally along the length of the vessel. Although the thickness of the adventitia will vary from vessel to vessel, in some muscular arteries it is equal in thickness to the media.

Figure 8-8 is a photomicrograph of a muscular artery stained specifically for elastin. Note the prominent *internal elastic membrane* and *external elastic membrane* within the wall of this vessel.

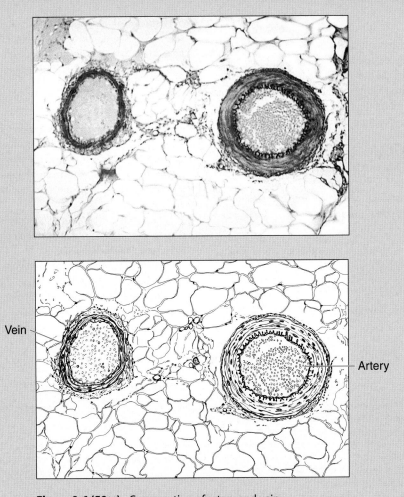

Vein

Artery

Figure 8-6 (50×): Cross section of artery and vein.

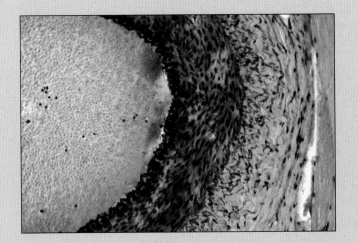

Figure 8-7 (100×): Cross section of a muscular artery.

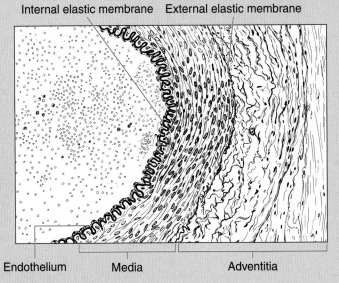

Internal elastic membrane   External elastic membrane

Endothelium   Media   Adventitia

Arterioles

Arterioles serve as the transition vessel between muscular arteries and capillaries. Three distinguishable coats (intima, media, and adventitia) are still evident in an arteriole.

Although a few, isolated elastic fibers may be seen in arterioles, an internal elastic membrane is not visible in small arterioles. In larger arterioles, however, a faint internal elastic membrane may be visible.

The media of an arteriole possesses only one or two layers of smooth muscle. The adventitia is thin and quite difficult to distinguish from any surrounding connective tissue.

Because of the difficulty and ambiguity in distinguishing between small and large arterioles, in this text an arteriole will be defined as a vessel that:

- Has the wall–thickness-to-lumen ratio that qualifies it as being a part of the arterial system

- Possesses one or two layers of smooth muscle

- Lacks an internal elastic membrane

Figure 8-9 demonstrates two *arterioles* within the adipose tissue that surrounds the pancreas. Close examination will show that these arterioles possess *one to two layers of smooth muscle* and lack an internal elastic membrane.

Capillaries

Figures 8-9 and **8-10** are photomicrographs of *capillaries* of varying diameters within adipose tissue. Note that the lumen diameter ranges in size from slightly smaller than a single red blood cell (RBC) to one and one-half times the diameter of an RBC.

The wall of a capillary has only one layer—the intima. The intima of a capillary is composed of one to three circumferentially arranged endothelial cells.

Because a capillary lacks a media, no smooth muscle cells will be found within its wall.

Note the sectioning and staining artifacts in the lower left corner of **Figure 8-10**.

Table 8-1: Summary of Histological Characteristics of Capillaries and Arteries

Blood Vessels	Intima	Media	Adventitia
Capillary	Single layer of endothelial cells and underlying subendothelial layer of loose (areolar) connective tissue	None present	None present
Arterioles	Endothelial cells and underlying connective tissue. Small arterioles lack an internal elastic membrane; larger arterioles may have a very delicate internal elastic membrane.	Only 1 to 2 layers of smooth muscle	Dense, irregular connective tissue composed of longitudinally and circumferentially arranged collagen and elastin fibers
Muscular artery	Endothelial cells on underlying connective tissue; internal elastic membrane present	Smooth muscle and some elastin and collagen; external elastic membrane present	Composed of longitudinally and circumferentially arranged collagen and elastin
Elastic artery	Relatively thick layer with endothelium on underlying connective tissue; internal elastic membrane present but not distinct because of numerous layers of elastic tissue within media	Thick layer of smooth muscle with fenestrated layers of elastin; external elastic membrane present but not distinct because of numerous layers of elastic tissue within media	Thin layer composed of collagen longitudinally arranged; often interspersed with elastic fibers

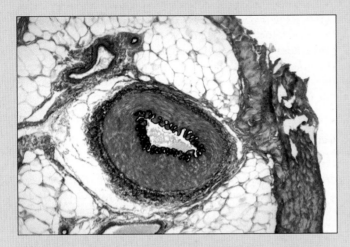

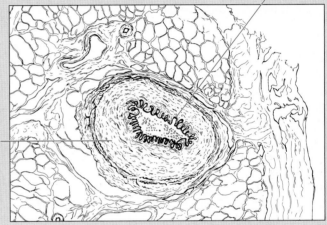

Figure 8-8 (100×): Cross section of a muscular artery, stained specifically for elastin.

Internal elastic membrane

External elastic membrane

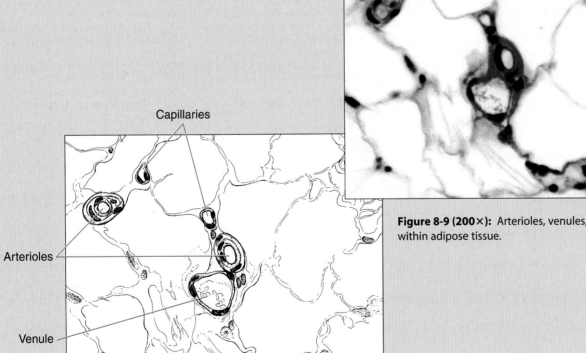

Capillaries

Arterioles

Venule

Figure 8-9 (200×): Arterioles, venules, and capillaries within adipose tissue.

Venous System

Vessels of the venous system possess the same three-layered organization as the arterial system. However, there are several histological characteristics of the venous system that easily distinguish its vessels from those of the arterial side of the cardiovascular system:

- The ratio of wall thickness to lumen diameter is considerably smaller for vessels of the venous system.

- The media is relatively thin and poorly developed in vessels of the venous system.

- Internal and external elastic membranes are more difficult to distinguish in vessels of the venous system.

Veins

Return to **Figure 8-6**. The vessel on the left is a vein. Use this photomicrograph to distinguish the histological differences between an artery and a vein. Note that the size of the lumen in both vessels is approximately equal. *However, the artery has a thicker wall than the vein. This wall–thickness-to-lumen ratio is a major feature to consider when trying to identify arteries and veins. An artery will always have a larger wall–thickness-to-lumen ratio than a vein of corresponding size.*

Keeping in mind the differences in the wall-to-lumen ratios between the two vessels in **Figure 8-6**, now examine the vein in the lower left corner of **Figure 8-11**. Only three to four layers of smooth muscle are seen within the media of this vein. You will also note that the *adventitia* and *intima* are more prominent in the vein as compared with that seen in an artery of comparable size (**Figure 8-7**).

Venules

Figures 8-9, 8-11, and **8-12** demonstrate the histology of an *arteriole* and *venule*. A venule is a transition vessel between a capillary and a vein. Because venules are part of the venous system, they have all of the histological characteristics of veins.

First, note the magnification of each photomicrograph. **Figure 8-11** demonstrates the relative size of an *arteriole* and *venule* compared with a *vein* and *muscular artery*, and **Figure 8-12** demonstrates the relative sizes of an *arteriole*, *capillary*, and *venule*.

Examination of **Figures 8-9** and **8-12** clearly demonstrates the wall-to-lumen ratio in arterioles and venules, as well as the thickness of the media of a venule. Both of these characteristics are major histological features of a venule.

Table 8-2: Summary of the Histology of the Cardiovascular System: Veins

Blood Vessel	Intima	Media	Adventitia
Venules	Endothelial cells on layer of areolar connective tissue	1 to 2 layers of smooth muscle	Relatively thick layer compared with intima or media
Veins: medium diameter	Layer composed of endothelium resting on subendothelial layer of thin collagen bundles interspersed with elastin. Internal elastic membrane present	Smooth muscle interspersed with elastic fibers that are often arranged longitudinally; external elastic membrane present but not prominent	Forms bulk of wall; composed of collagen and elastin and some longitudinally arranged smooth muscle fibers
Veins: large diameter	Similar to that of medium-diameter veins.	Poorly developed layer; collagen and some elastic fibers interspersed between smooth muscle	Relatively thick layer; bundles of irregularly arranged collagen and elastic fibers interspersed with longitudinally arranged smooth muscle

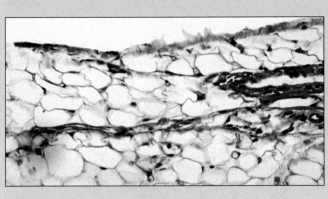

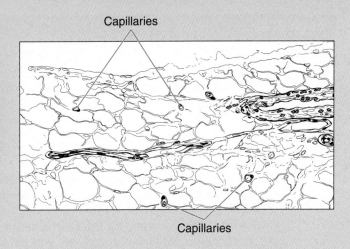

Capillaries

Figure 8-10 (200×): Capillaries within adipose tissue.

Capillaries

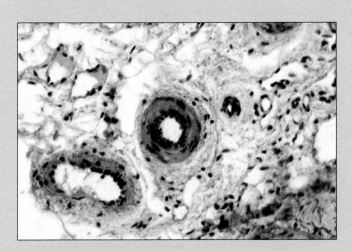

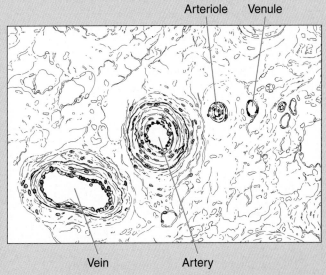

Arteriole   Venule

Figure 8-11 (200×): Cross section of a vein.

Vein   Artery

Capillaries

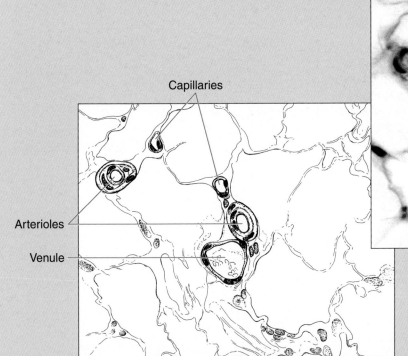

Arterioles

Venule

Figure 8-12 (200×): Cross section of venule and arteriole.

Logic Tree

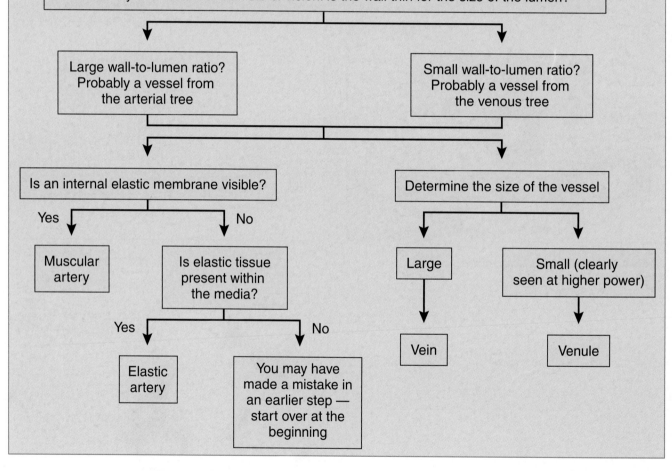

LOGIC TREE FOR BLOOD VESSELS

First determine the size of the vessel. Make a general distinction between larger (artery, vein) and smaller (arteriole, venule, capillary) vessels.

Once you have determined the size of the vessel you need to determine the wall-to-lumen ratio. If possible, scan the entire slide to find another vessel of comparable size but with a different wall-to-lumen ratio. Such a comparison will aid you in determining the wall-to-lumen ratio for the vessel in question. However, as you become more efficient in your identification process you will find that you can make this determination with only one vessel in the field of vision. Is the wall thin for the size of the lumen?

Large wall-to-lumen ratio? Probably a vessel from the arterial tree

Small wall-to-lumen ratio? Probably a vessel from the venous tree

Is an internal elastic membrane visible?

Yes → Muscular artery

No → Is elastic tissue present within the media?

Yes → Elastic artery

No → You may have made a mistake in an earlier step — start over at the beginning

Determine the size of the vessel

Large → Vein

Small (clearly seen at higher power) → Venule

BLOOD

Red Blood Cells and Platelets

Red blood cells (RBCs) (red blood cells or erythrocytes) are anucleated, biconcave cells that perform their major functions within the blood vessels of the cardiovascular system. **Figure 9-1** is an oil-immersion photomicrograph demonstrating red blood cells and platelets. Some of the *red blood cells* stain quite homogeneously, whereas a few may show a pale center. Other than this minor staining difference, red blood cells are unremarkable. *Platelets* are also visible as small purple dots between the RBCs in this photomicrograph.

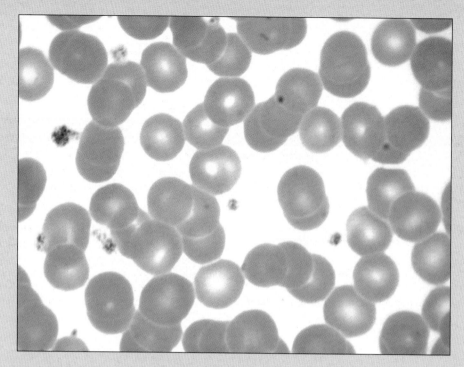

Figure 9-1 (350×): Red blood cells and platelets (Wright stain).

Leukocytes

Leukocytes (white blood cells) migrate out of the blood vessels to perform their functions (see Table 9-1). Unlike erythrocytes, leukocytes are nucleated blood cells that are subdivided into two groups on the basis of the presence *(granulocytes)* or absence *(agranulocytes)* of granules within their cytoplasms. Lymphocytes and monocytes are classified as agranulocytes, whereas neutrophils, basophils, and eosinophils are classified as granulocytes.

Table 9-1: Comparison of Blood Cells

Cell	Cells per μl	Major Function
Erythrocyte	$4.5\text{-}6.5 \times 10^6$	Transport of oxygen and carbon dioxide
Leukocyte (WBC)	$4\text{-}11 \times 10^3$	Defense mechanisms
Neutrophilic granulocytes	50%-70% of total WBC count	First white blood cell to arrive at the site of an infection in any large numbers; phagocytose antigens
Eosinophilic granulocyte	1%-4% of total WBC count	Release of histamines in inflammatory reactions
Basophilic granulocyte	Less than 1% of total WBC count	Involved in acute inflammation and allergic reactions by releasing histamine and interleukins
Monocyte	2%-8% of total WBC count	Migrate to sites of infection in large numbers; able to leave the bloodstream and ingest bacteria and cellular debris. Are termed macrophages when they exit the cardiovascular system and enter the extracellular space.
Lymphocyte	20%-40% of total WBC count	Appear at infection site at approximately the same time as monocytes. Some transform into plasmocytes. Only WBC able to recognize specific antigens and only WBC with an immunological memory.

WBC, White blood cell.

Agranulocytes

Lymphocyte

Lymphocytes (Figure 9-2) are the second most common cell type among the leukocytes, with neutrophils being the most common. (See Table 9-1.) The most obvious feature of a lymphocyte is a rounded nucleus that contains a small dimple on one side. A rim of cytoplasm surrounds the nucleus, which is variable in both amount and staining characteristics, depending on the size of the lymphocyte.

Monocytes

Monocytes (Figure 9-3) are not as numerous as lymphocytes. The cell is quite large and possesses a rather blue-gray, irregularly staining cytoplasm. The nucleus will vary from kidney shaped to horseshoe shaped and is usually mottled in appearance.

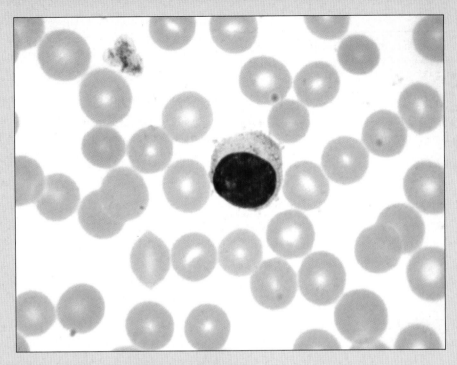

Figure 9-2 (350×): Lymphocyte (Wright stain).

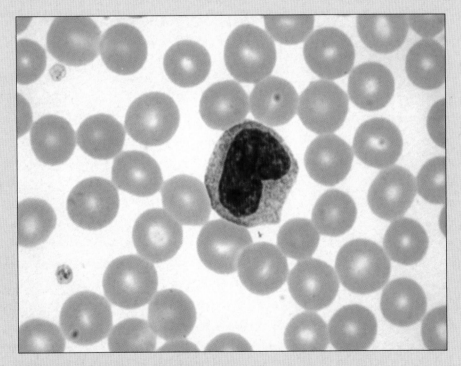

Figure 9-3 (350×): Monocyte (Wright stain).

Granulocytes

Granulocytes are subdivided into different categories according to (1) the presence or absence of cytoplasmic granules, (2) the staining properties of those granules, and (3) the shape of the nucleus of the cell. *Because the cytoplasmic granules of eosinophils and basophils often obscure the nucleus from view, it is best to base your identification mostly on the staining properties of the cytoplasmic granules, if they are present.*

Eosinophilic Granulocyte

Eosinophilic granulocytes (eosinophils) have a bilobed nucleus, with each lobe being quite smooth in outline and approximately the same size (**Figure 9-4**). The cytoplasm contains rather large, eosinophilic granules. In some eosinophils (such as the one in this photomicrograph), the granules are so prominent that they obscure some or all of the nucleus from view.

Basophilic Granulocyte

Basophilic granulocytes (basophils) (**Figure 9-5**) are quite rare in a normal blood smear. Such cells contain a bilobed nucleus and prominent basophilic cytoplasmic granules, which normally obscure the nucleus from view.

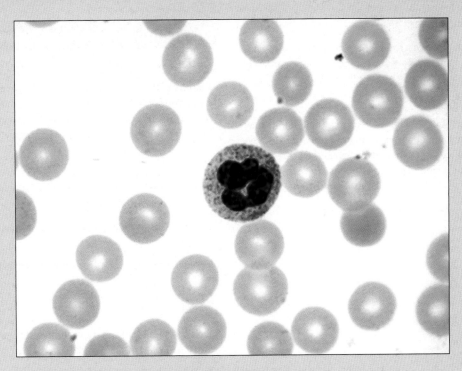

Figure 9-4 (350×): Eosinophilic granulocyte (Wright stain).

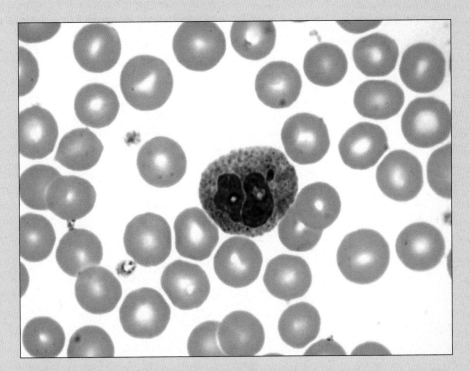

Figure 9-5 (350×): Basophilic granulocyte (Wright stain).

Neutrophilic Granulocytes

Neutrophilic granulocytes (neutrophils) are by far the most numerous leukocytes (Figure 9-6). Neutrophils are approximately the same size as basophilic and eosinophilic granulocytes. Neutrophils contain a segmented nucleus and have a relatively clear cytoplasm because the granules are just at or below the resolution of the light microscope. The nucleus of a neutrophil may possess as few as two segments or as many as six. These segments, which are joined together by thin strands of chromatin, are quite irregular in shape. *The shape of the nucleus and the relatively clear cytoplasm both serve as excellent histological characteristics.*

Commonly Misidentified Tissues

Monocytes and Large Lymphocytes

Assuming that the granules found in neutrophils, basophils, and eosinophils stain normally, thereby minimizing identification errors, the two blood cells that are most commonly misidentified are the monocyte and lymphocyte.

Monocyte (Review **Figure 9-3** in section on Monocytes)

1. Is the larger of the two cells in question (approximately 12 to 15 μM in diameter).

2. Possesses more cytoplasm. Cytoplasm stains blue/gray in color.

3. Nucleus usually possesses noticeable indentation.

Lymphocyte (Review **Figure 9-2** in section on Lymphocytes)

1. Is the smaller of the two cells in question (approximately 10 to 12 μM in diameter).

2. Has slightly less cytoplasm, often seen as a thin rim around the nucleus. Cytoplasm stains blue in color.

3. Nucleus is more rounded. If indentation is present, it is considerably less prominent in the large lymphocyte.

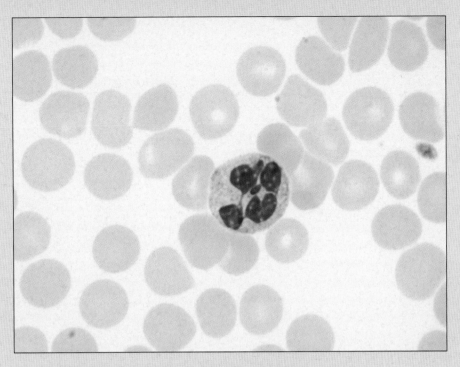

Figure 9-6 (350×): Neutrophilic granulocyte (Wright stain).

Chapter 10

RESPIRATORY SYSTEM

Chapter Objectives

This chapter will enable you to:

1. Discuss and identify the forms of epithelium found from the trachea to the alveoli.

2. Identify each subdivision of the respiratory tree from the trachea to the alveoli.

3. Identify pneumocyte type I cells, pneumocyte type II cells, and alveolar macrophages within the alveoli of the lung.

Characteristics of the Conducting and Exchange Portions of the Respiratory System

The respiratory system is subdivided into conducting and exchange pathways. These pathways demonstrate structural specializations that facilitate (1) the conditioning of the air (warming, moistening, and cleaning) within the conducting pathway and (2) gas exchange with the cardiovascular system within the exchange pathway.

The conducting pathways of the respiratory system are those areas that are not anatomically designed for gas exchange. These pathways consist of the nasal cavities, pharynx, larynx, trachea, bronchi, and terminal bronchioles. (Only the histology of the conducting pathway from the trachea to the terminal bronchioles is discussed in this chapter.) The ability of these pathways to condition the air is accomplished by distinct histological characteristics:

- Hyaline cartilage is present, in varying forms, in all conducting pathways except bronchioles. Hyaline cartilage helps to maintain the patency of the conducting pathways.

- Seromucous glands are found in all conducting pathways except terminal bronchioles. These glands help to moisten and lubricate the conducting pathways and trap foreign particles.

- Mucous cells are found in all conducting pathways except terminal bronchioles. These cells produce mucus, which helps to moisten and lubricate the conducting pathways and trap foreign particles.

- Cilia are found within the conducting pathways wherever mucous cells are present. Cilia help to remove mucus produced by mucous cells.

- Elastic fibers are found in the subepithelial connective tissue of all conducting pathways except the nose. Elastic fibers help to maintain the patency of the conducting pathways.

- The conducting pathways demonstrate the classic respiratory epithelium (ciliated pseudostratified columnar) at every level except the bronchioles.

- All conducting pathways possess a high degree of vascularity.

The exchange portion of the respiratory system starts at the level of the respiratory bronchioles—the level at which alveoli make their first appearance. Alveoli are specialized for gas exchange. The shape of the squamous epithelium provides a large surface area and a thin diffusion barrier. The exchange portion of the respiratory system is marked by a high degree of vascularity. Three cell types are found within the exchange portion of the respiratory system:

- Pneumocyte Type I cells (also termed *squamous alveolar cells* or *septal cells*):

  - Are squamous in shape and form a simple squamous epithelium, thereby providing a minimal diffusion barrier between the alveolus and surrounding capillaries

  - Occupy approximately 95% of the alveolar surface

- Pneumocyte Type II cells (also termed *great alveolar cells*):

  - Demonstrate an irregular cuboidal shape

  - Occupy approximately 5% of the alveolar surface

  - Produce surfactant

- Alveolar macrophages (dust cells):

  - Are freely wandering phagocytic cells that are not part of the alveolar wall but are often found sitting on the alveolar surface

  - Are derived from circulating monocytes

Trachea

Some histological slides of the trachea also contain a cross section of the esophagus. Scan the section at low power first and then proceed to a higher magnification after you have distinguished the trachea from the esophagus.

Figures 10-1 and 10-2 clearly demonstrate that the *epithelium of the trachea* is a ciliated, pseudostratified, columnar epithelium with mucous cells. (See sections on the Pseudostratified Ciliated Columnar Epithelium and Unicellular Exocrine Glands in Chapter 2.) The epithelium rests on a prominent connective tissue layer termed the *lamina propria*. This epithelium possesses three distinctively different cell types (not all of which are visible in this photomicrograph): mucous cells, tall ciliated cells, and short (stem) cells.

The lamina propria contains numerous elastic fibers that cannot be seen in standard hematoxylin and eosin (H & E) preparations. The *submucosa* is loose, irregular (areolar) connective tissue containing *mixed tubuloacinar seromucous glands* and adipose cells (see sections on Loose, Irregular [Areolar] Connective Tissue and Adipose Tissue in Chapter 3).

The framework and chief support of the trachea is composed of *C-shaped hyaline cartilage* (see section on Hyaline Cartilage in Chapter 4). Depending on the plane of section, the cartilage may not be in a complete C-shape. The posterior, open portions of the cartilage are joined by fibroelastic connective tissue and smooth muscle (see section on Smooth Muscle in Chapter 6).

Table 10-1: Histological Characteristics of the Respiratory System

Region	Epithelium	Mucous Cells	Glands	Cartilage	Smooth Muscle	Elastic Fibers
Nasal cavity	Pseudostratified columnar*	Large number	Large number	Hyaline	None	None
Larynx	Pseudostratified columnar†	Large number	Large number	Complex: hyaline and elastic	None	Yes
Trachea	Pseudostratified columnar	Large number	Yes	C-shaped hyaline cartilage	Yes	Yes
Small bronchi	Pseudostratified columnar	Few	Few	Plates and islands	Cross-spiral layers	Yes
Terminal bronchioles	Simple low columnar or cuboidal; ciliated	None	None	None	Cross-spiral layers	Yes
Respiratory bronchioles	Simple cuboidal, ciliated proximally, not distally	None	None	None	Cross-spiral layers	Yes
Alveolar ducts	Simple squamous, nonciliated	None	None	None	Yes‡	Yes
Alveoli	Simple squamous (type I) or simple cuboidal (type II)	None	None	None	Yes‡	Yes

* Stratified squamous epithelium in regions of direct airflow or abrasion.
† Vestibule shows transition from stratified squamous epithelium with keratin to characteristic epithelium of the respiratory system.
‡ Concentrated at alveolar openings.

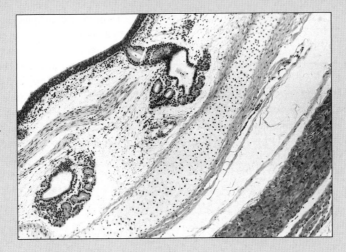

Figure 10-1 (25×): Trachea.

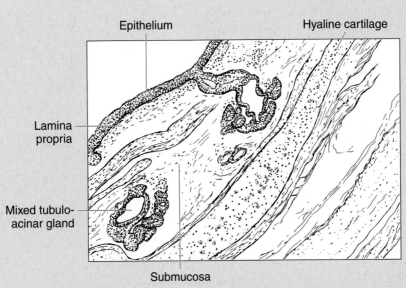

Epithelium

Hyaline cartilage

Lamina
propria

Mixed tubulo-
acinar gland

Submucosa

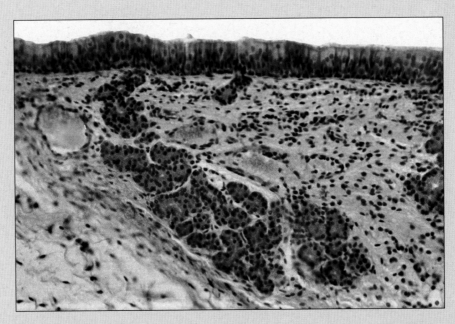

Figure 10-2 (50×): Trachea.

Lung

Bronchi

Figures 10-3 and 10-4 show a bronchus within a human lung. The surfaces of the lungs are covered with a serous membrane called the *visceral pleura*, which is continuous with the parietal pleura at the hilus. The visceral pleura may or may not be visible on your sections. It is not visible on either of these figures.

The main bronchus will divide into secondary bronchi after entering the lung. The *hyaline cartilage* of the larger bronchi will form complete rings as compared with the C-shaped cartilage seen in the trachea. In smaller bronchi, the rings give way to irregular plates and islands of hyaline cartilage.

The wall of a *bronchus* is continuous, and its *epithelium* is a typical respiratory epithelium: pseudostratified, columnar epithelium with cilia and mucous cells. Large bundles of *smooth muscle* will be seen intertwined with elastic fibers within the wall of the bronchus. *Bronchial glands* are present in the bronchial walls in numbers equal to or greater than those seen in the trachea. These bronchial glands may be serous, mucous, or seromucous in nature (see section on Epithelial Glands in Chapter 2).

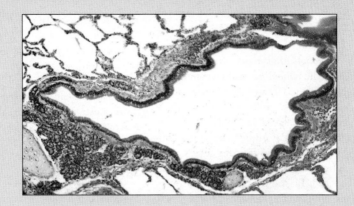

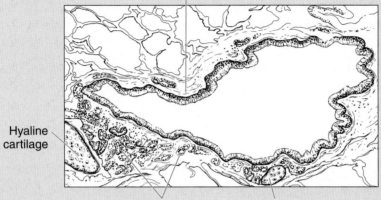

Smooth muscle

Hyaline
cartilage

Bronchial glands   Hyaline cartilage

Figure 10-3 (25×): Bronchus.

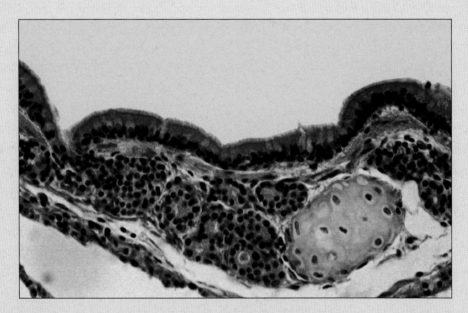

Figure 10-4 (50×): Bronchus.

Terminal and Respiratory Bronchioles

Figure 10-5 illustrates the transition from a terminal bronchiole to a respiratory bronchiole. *Terminal bronchioles* are characterized by their *continuous walls*. The *epithelium* will change from a typical respiratory epithelium proximally to a simple columnar epithelium in the more distal segments, followed by a simple cuboidal epithelium in the most distal portions (see section on Simple Cuboidal Epithelia in Chapter 2). All of these epithelial variations possess cilia. The epithelium lacks mucous cells.

The lamina propria in a terminal bronchiole is rather thick, as is the amount of smooth muscle. Elastic fibers, which are not visible in H & E preparations, are found in higher proportions in terminal bronchioles than in bronchi. Cartilage and seromucous glands are absent from the walls of a terminal bronchiole.

The walls of *respiratory bronchioles* are discontinuous because of the presence of *pulmonary alveoli* in their walls. Between the alveoli, this subdivision of the respiratory system is lined by a *simple cuboidal epithelium*. This epithelium of a respiratory bronchiole is rather tall at the more proximal regions and considerably lower in height in the more distal portions. Cilia are present in the more proximal portions but will be absent in the distal portions.

Smooth muscle and elastic fibers are prominent in the walls of the respiratory bronchioles.

As was seen in terminal bronchioles, cartilage and seromucous glands are absent within the walls of a respiratory bronchiole.

A question to consider: What is the anatomical and physiological rationale for the presence of cilia in regions of the respiratory tree lacking in mucous cells and glands?

Alveoli

Figure 10-6 shows a respiratory bronchiole terminating at an *alveolar duct*, which in turn terminates in *alveoli*. The walls of an alveolar duct are formed by pulmonary sacs and alveoli. Only a few *simple squamous* to *low cuboidal cells* (see section on Simple Squamous Epithelia in Chapter 2) may be found in the walls between the alveoli. Smooth muscle cells are concentrated around the alveolar openings but are not visible in these sections. Reticular, elastic, and delicate collagenous fibers are also present but not visible.

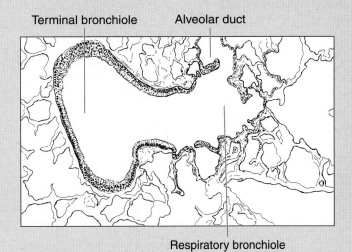

Terminal bronchiole   Alveolar duct

Respiratory bronchiole

Figure 10-5 (50×): Transition from a terminal bronchiole to a respiratory bronchiole.

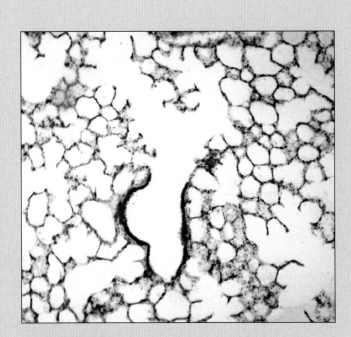

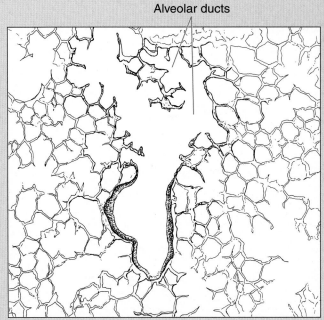

Alveolar ducts

Figure 10-6 (25×): Alveolar duct.

The *alveoli* (Figure 10-7) are lined by *pneumocyte type I* cells (also termed *squamous alveolar cells*), *pneumocyte type II* cells (also termed *great alveolar cells* or *septal cells*), and alveolar macrophages (also termed dust cells). Alveolar macrophages are difficult to identify with the light microscope unless they have ingested foreign particles.

The rich capillary networks of the lungs are fed by pulmonary arteries, the larger of which are usually seen in close proximity to bronchi and bronchioles. The capillaries drain into small pulmonary veins that course through the connective tissue septa between lung lobules. The larger pulmonary arteries run along the bronchioles opposite the corresponding pulmonary veins. Bronchiolar arteries may also be seen in some of your slide preparations. They are typically smaller in diameter than pulmonary arteries. What is the function of each of these types of vessels?

Commonly Misidentified Tissues

Artery and Small Bronchiole

At low or medium power a beginning student in histology may confuse a small bronchiole and a blood vessel, usually an artery. Therefore it is important to keep the following differences in mind:

Artery (Review **Figures 8-6** to **8-8** in section on Muscular Arteries in Chapter 8)

1. Presence of Red Blood Cells (RBCs) in lumen

2. Thin, convoluted layer of tissue lining lumen; simple squamous epithelium on connective tissue upon close examination

3. Prominent outer layer (adventitia) composed of connective tissue

4. Thick layer of smooth muscle

Small Bronchiole (Review **Figure 10-5** in section on Terminal and Respiratory Bronchioles)

1. Clear lumen

2. Prominent folds in the thick epithelium lining wall of tubule; epithelium pseudostratified columnar with cilia and mucous cells upon close examination

3. Thin layer of smooth muscle

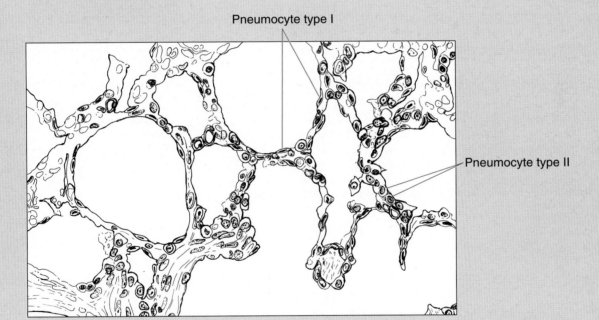

Pneumocyte type I

Pneumocyte type II

Figure 10-7 (100×): Pulmonary alveoli.

Logic Tree

LOGIC TREE FOR THE RESPIRATORY SYSTEM

Because many structures within the respiratory system branch into distal structures within the same field of vision it is very important to look first for histological features *only in the designated region.* Looking at too wide of a field of vision may lead to a misidentification.

Is the wall of the unknown structure continuous?

Yes — No

Yes branch:

Is cartilage present in the wall of the structure?

No — Yes

No (cartilage): Simple columnar or simple cuboidal epithelium?

- Simple columnar → Terminal bronchiole
- Simple cuboidal → Identification error

Yes (cartilage): Pseudostratified columnar epithelium with cilia and mucous cells?

- No → Identification error
- Yes → Tubuloacinar glands present?
  - Yes → Trachea
  - No → Identification error*

No branch:

Is cartilage present in the wall of the structure?

No — Yes

No (cartilage): Simple cuboidal or simple squamous epithelium?

- Simple cuboidal → Respiratory bronchiole
- Simple squamous → Alveolar duct

Yes (cartilage): Identification error

*Note: Some sections of trachea may not demonstrate tubuloacinar glands.

Chapter 11

LYMPHOID SYSTEM

Chapter Objectives

This chapter will enable you to identify:

1. Lymphoid nodules

2. Various types of lymphoid organs

3. Various forms of lymphoid tissue of mucous membranes

4. Various cells typically found within all forms of lymphoid tissue

Lymphatic tissue is a specialized form of epithelial and connective tissue that is regularly infiltrated with lymphocytes. Lymphocytes will be distributed throughout the body in a variety of ways, including:

- Individual, encapsulated lymphoid organs

- Nonencapsulated lymphoid nodules within connective tissue

- Isolated aggregates of lymphoid cells

Diffuse Lymphoid Tissue and Lymphoid Nodules

Diffuse Lymphoid Tissue

Diffuse lymphoid tissue may be found within various portions of the respiratory, urogenital, and digestive systems. **Figure 11-1** demonstrates *diffuse lymphoid tissue* in close association with a bronchus of the respiratory system. What would be an advantage of having lymphoid tissue in this region of the respiratory system?

Lymphoid Nodules

Lymphoid nodules, which are typically oval in shape, are aggregations of lymphocytes contained within a supporting framework of reticular fibers. There are two forms of lymphoid nodules: primary and secondary. A primary nodule is composed almost exclusively of small lymphocytes. Most lymphoid nodules, however, are secondary nodules. Secondary nodules have the following histological characteristics:

- An outer ring of small, dark-staining lymphocytes

- An inner, lighter-staining region termed a *germinal center* that contains larger, paler-staining lymphocytes

Aggregated Lymphoid Nodules (Peyer's Patches)

Aggregated lymphatic nodules (also termed *Peyer's Patches*) **(Figure 11-2)** are groups of lymphoid nodules found in the ileum of the small intestine, especially near its junction with the colon. They always occur on the side of the gut opposite the attachment of the mesentery.

Each group of aggregated lymphoid nodules consists of 10 to 70 nodules lying side by side and arranged such that the entire group has an oval shape, with its long diameter lying lengthwise in the intestine. The apices of the nodules are pear shaped and directed toward the lumen. They almost project through the entire thickness of the mucosa.

The surface of the small intestine is lacking villi at the location of the nodules. As you look at **Figure 11-2**, it appears that villi are indeed present on the intestinal surface at the location of the aggregated lymphoid nodules. What good histological reason could be given for the apparent presence of villi immediately superficial to the location of aggregated lymphoid nodules?

Lymphoid Organs

Palatine Tonsil

Figure 11-3 shows a palatine tonsil covered with a *nonkeratinized, stratified squamous epithelium (mucosal type)* (see section on Stratified Squamous Epithelium in Chapter 2). The stratified squamous epithelium is continuous with the free surface of the pharynx. At various locations on the surface of the tonsil, deep indentations or pockets, termed *crypts* (not visible on this photomicrograph), will occur. Distributed along the crypts are *lymphoid nodules*. Many of these nodules will possess *germinal centers*.

Pharyngeal Tonsil

Pharyngeal tonsils **(Figure 11-4)** are quite similar to palatine tonsils. However, the epithelium on the free surface is different because it is composed of a *typical respiratory epithelium* (pseudostratified columnar epithelium with cilia and mucous cells) (see section on Pseudostratified Ciliated Columnar Epithelium in Chapter 2). Patches of stratified squamous epithelium are sometimes found on pharyngeal tonsils of humans, more commonly on the pharyngeal tonsils of a child than on those of an adult.

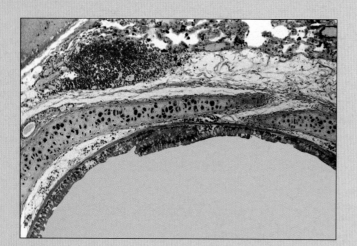

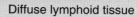
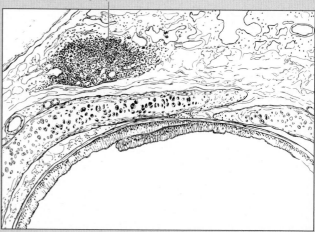

Figure 11-1 (25×): Diffuse lymphoid tissue associated within a bronchus of the respiratory system.

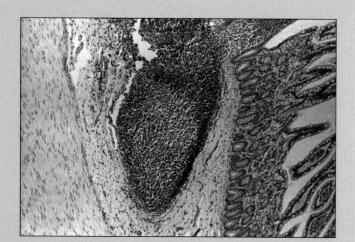

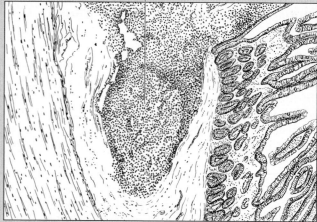

Figure 11-2 (25×): Palatine tonsil.

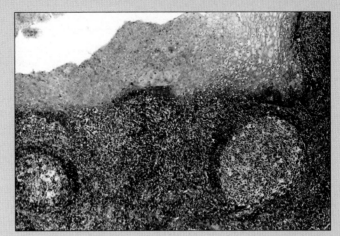

Figure 11-3 (25×): Palatine tonsil.

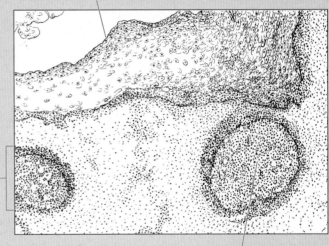

Stratified squamous epithelium

Lymphoid
nodule

Germinal
center

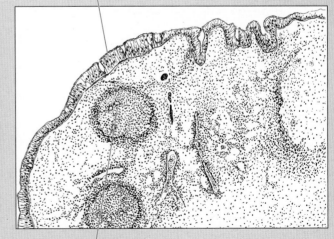

Respiratory epithelium

Figure 11-4 (25×): Pharyngeal tonsil.

Lymphoid nodule
with germinal center

Lymph Nodes

Lymph nodes are small, encapsulated lymphoid organs found along the course of lymphatic vessels throughout the body. Figure 11-5 is a line drawing of a lymph node. Use this figure to orientate yourself to the following structures of a lymph node:

- Lymph nodes are covered with a connective tissue capsule of collagenous fibers, scattered elastic fibers, and smooth muscle cells.

- At various regions of the node, the capsule extends into the body of the organ as trabeculae.

- Lymph nodes will possess several afferent lymph vessels and only one or two efferent lymph vessels.

- Lymph nodes are divided into an outer cortex and an inner medulla.

Figure 11-6 demonstrates how, at various regions of the organ, the connective tissue *capsule* extends into the body of the organ as *trabeculae*. Immediately deep to the capsule you will find the first of a series of an interconnected system of spaces, termed the *subcapsular space* (also called the *subcapsular sinus* or *marginal sinus*). The subcapsular space is continuous, with a space found on either side of the trabeculae, termed the *paratrabecular* space (also termed *trabecular sinuses*, *intermediate sinuses* or *cortical sinuses*), which may not be visible on your section.

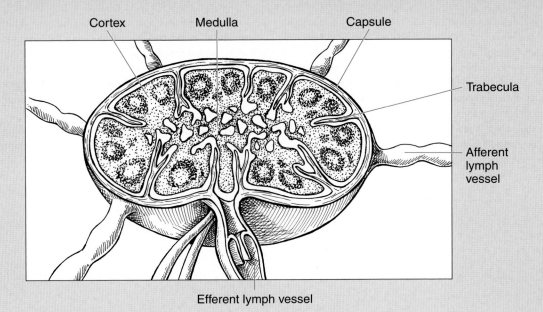

Figure 11-5 Line drawing of a lymph node.

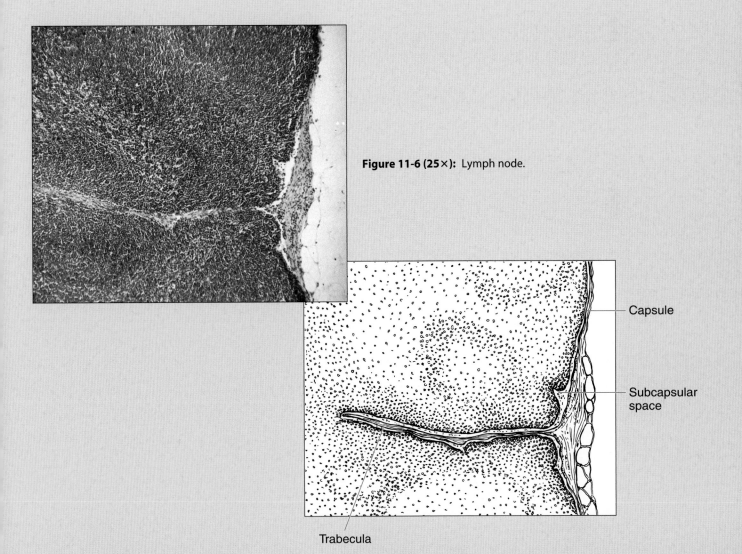

Figure 11-6 (25×): Lymph node.

Figure 11-7 demonstrates that the trabeculae and elements of the lymphoid organ are arranged differently in the outer (cortical) and inner (medullary) regions of the organ.

In the *cortex*, the trabeculae are arranged more or less perpendicular to the surface. The lymphocytes of the cortex are closely packed, forming nodules. If these nodules are composed mostly of small lymphocytes, they are termed *primary nodules*. However, if they possess a paler central zone, called a *germinal center*, they are termed *secondary nodules*.

The *deep cortex* (also termed the *juxtamedullary cortex* or *paracortex*) lacks nodules, and the cells are more loosely packed than those within the more superficial cortex. Small lymphocytes are the most common cell type within the deep cortex, and large lymphocytes, plasmocytes, and macrophages are rarely seen. **Figure 11-8** demonstrates the cortex of a lymph node, including *primary* and *secondary* nodules.

The *medulla* of the lymph node is composed of *medullary cords* surrounded by medullary sinuses. The medullary cords are

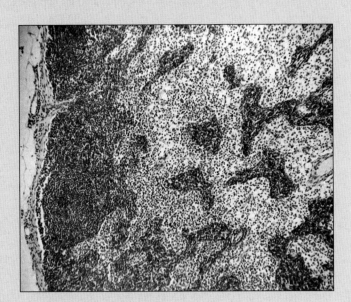

Figure 11-7 (25×): Lymph node.

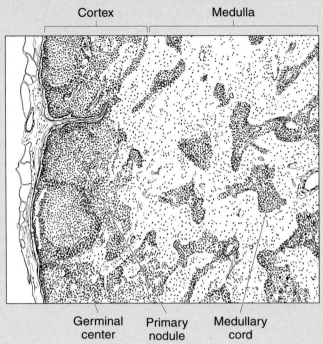

Cortex   Medulla

Germinal   Primary   Medullary
center   nodule   cord

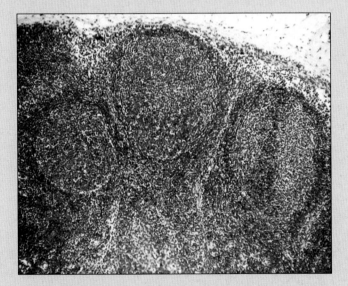

Figure 11-8 (25×): Lymph node.

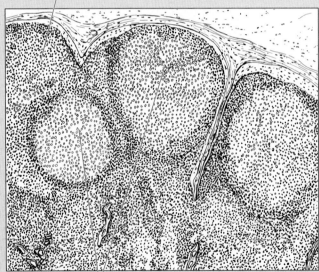

Primary
nodule

Secondary nodule
with germinal center

aggregations of lymphoid tissue. These cords branch and anastomose freely and are not prominent in a resting lymph node. They are composed of reticular fibers, reticular cells, small lymphocytes, plasmocytes, and macrophages. **Figure 11-9** demonstrates a cross-sectional view and a longitudinal view of *medullary sinuses*. These sinuses are surrounded by lymphocytes arranged into poorly defined medullary cords.

Reticular cells, macrophages, and endothelial cells line the medullary sinuses. Medullary sinuses, which are continuous with the subscapular and paratrabecular spaces, are lined by reticular cells and macrophages. Gaps between adjacent endothelial cells (not visible on the photomicrograph) in medullary sinuses are considerably larger than the gaps in the capillaries of the cardiovascular system.

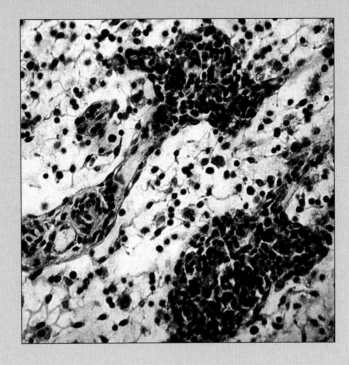

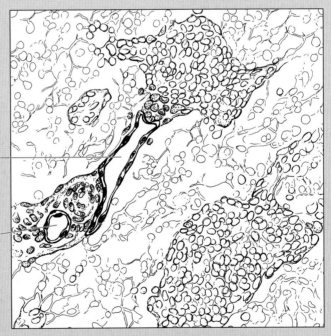

Medullary sinus
longitudinal section

Medullary sinus
cross section

Figure 11-9 (100×): Medullary sinuses of a lymph node.

Thymus

Thymus/Child

The thymus is composed of lobules joined by connective tissue and slender strands of lymphoid tissue. A *capsule* composed of fibroelastic connective tissue surrounds the gland. Relatively coarse *trabeculae* branch off of the capsule and incompletely divide the gland into lobules.

Figure 11-10 shows that each lobule of the thymus contains a cortex and medulla. The *cortex* of the thymus stains more basophilic as compared with the *medulla*. This staining differential is due to the varying cellular populations in the cortex and medulla, in that thymic lymphocytes are found in higher concentrations within the cortex as compared with the medulla.

The thymus *lacks lymphoid nodules; this is a major histological feature.*

Throughout the entire thymus are epithelioreticular cells (not visible in this photomicrograph), the second cell type found within the thymus. Epithelioreticular cells are actually epithelial cells joined to one another by desmosomes at the end of long, cytoplasmic processes. These epithelioreticular cells serve as a cellular framework for the thymus and histologically resemble reticular cells.

Thymic corpuscles (also termed *Hassal's corpuscles*) are visible in Figures 11-10 and 11-11. *These structures, which are major histological features of the thymus,* are composed of concentrically arranged epithelioreticular cells. Their function is unknown.

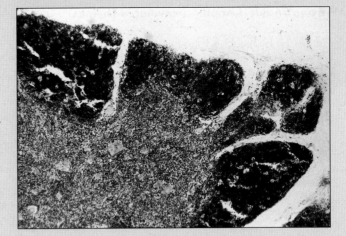

Figure 11-10 (25×): Thymus of a child.

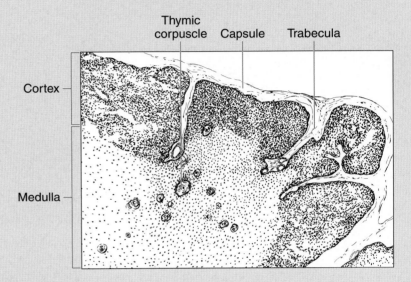

Thymic corpuscle   Capsule   Trabecula

Cortex —

Medulla —

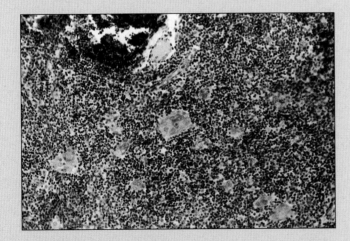

Figure 11-11 (50×): Thymus of a child.

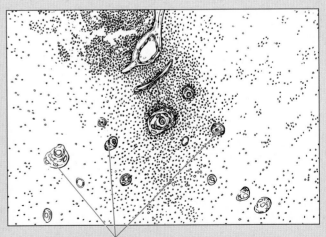

Thymic corpuscles

Thymus/Adult (Atrophic or Involuted Thymus)

Figures 11-12 and 11-13 show an adult thymus undergoing atrophy or involution, which is believed to start at puberty. However, a relative decline in the volume of thymic parenchyma may actually begin earlier in childhood.

During the involution process, the thymus is infiltrated with adipose tissue. The clearly lobulated structure, as well as the definitive medullary and cortical structure, is lost. The number of thymic lymphocytes is reduced, and the epithelioreticular cell becomes the major cellular element. *Thymic (Hassal's) corpuscles, however, are not affected by the involution process and remain a major histological feature of the thymus, regardless of the age of the individual from whom the specimen was obtained.*

Compare the features exhibited in an atrophic thymus to those of a thymus from a healthy child (see Figures 11-10 and 11-11).

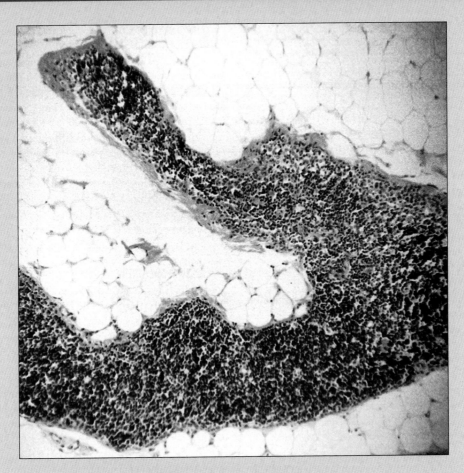

Figure 11-12 (25×): Atrophic thymus.

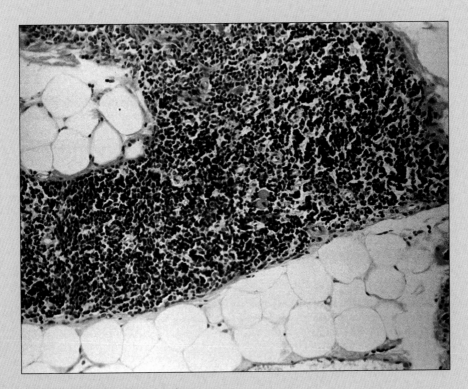

Figure 11-13 (50×): Atrophic thymus.

Spleen

The spleen (Figure 11-14) is covered by a fibrous capsule that possesses numerous elastic fibers and some smooth muscle. (The capsule is not visible on this photomicrograph.) Dense *trabeculae* extend into the spleen from the capsule. These will branch and form incomplete anastomosing chambers. Located adjacent to or within the trabeculae are *trabecular arteries* and *trabecular veins*.

The spaces between the connective tissue trabeculae are filled with soft, spongy tissue known as *splenic pulp* (Figure 11-15). On the basis of color differences seen in freshly dissected preparations, the pulp is subdivided into *red pulp* (also called *splenic cords*) and *white pulp* (also called *lymphoid nodules*). *Red and white pulp will not stain red and white in your preparations*, nor do they appear red and white in these photomicrographs. Both types of pulp are composed of lymphoid tissue.

The white pulp (Figure 11-16) consists of lymphocytes. In hematoxylin and eosin sections, white pulp stains basophilic because of the presence of numerous lymphocyte nuclei. The white pulp of the spleen is aggregated into *lymphoid nodules*. These nodules contain *germinal centers,* which tend to decrease in number with increasing age. Within each germinal center is a *central arteriole* (previously termed a *central artery*) that is a continuation of the trabecular artery. This central arteriole may be centrally located within the germinal center, or it may be displaced peripherally. *Regardless of its location, the presence of a central arteriole associated with a lymphoid nodule is a major histological feature of the spleen.*

Figure 11-17 demonstrates a lymphoid nodule with a germinal center on the right side of the photomicrograph. Figure 11-18 is a high-power photomicrograph of the red pulp found adjacent to the lymphoid nodule seen in Figure 11-17.

Surrounding the white pulp is a diffuse cellular network that constitutes the *red pulp* of the spleen (Figures 11-17 and 11-18). The red pulp consists of *venous sinuses* (also termed *splenic sinuses*) surrounded by splenic cords (the cords of Billroth). Splenic cords consist of reticular fibers and reticular cells supporting lymphocytes, macrophages, plasmocytes, erythrocytes, and various granulocytes (see sections on Loose, Irregular Connective Tissue [Mesenteric Spread] and Loose, Irregular Connective Tissue [Lamina Propria of the Duodenum] in Chapter 3).

Endothelial cells (Figure 11-18) line the venous sinuses of the red pulp. The sinuses are extremely attenuated and orientated with their axis parallel to the longitudinal axis of the sinus. The large spaces between these endothelial cells facilitate the easy passage of erythrocytes into and out of the sinuses.

Appendix

The appendix is often classified as a lymphoid organ. However, it will be discussed in conjunction with the hollow organs of the gastrointestinal tract in Chapter 16.

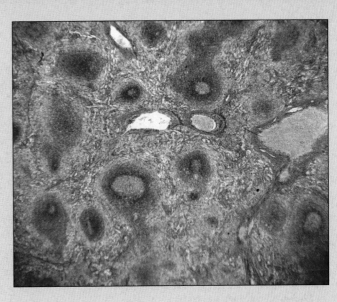

Figure 11-14 (50×): Spleen.

Trabecular vein

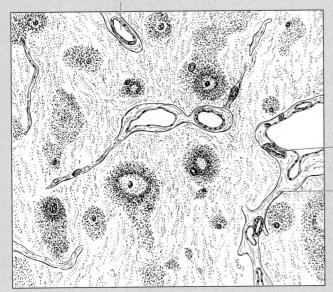

Trabecular artery

Trabecula

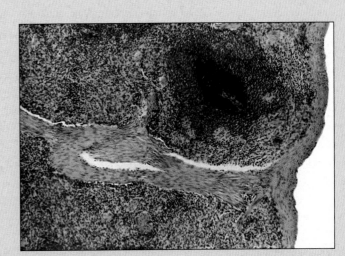

Figure 11-15 (25×): Spleen.

Capsule

Red pulp
(splenic cords)

White pulp
(lymphoid nodule)

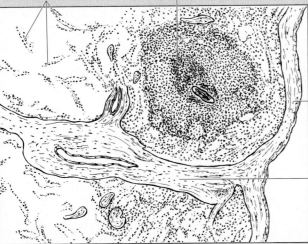

Trabecula

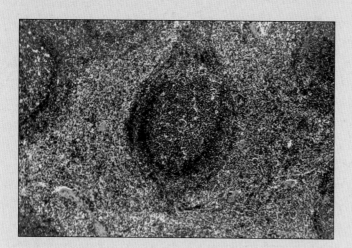

Figure 11-16 (50×): Spleen.

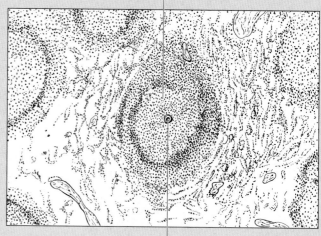

Lymphoid nodule with germinal center

Central arteriole

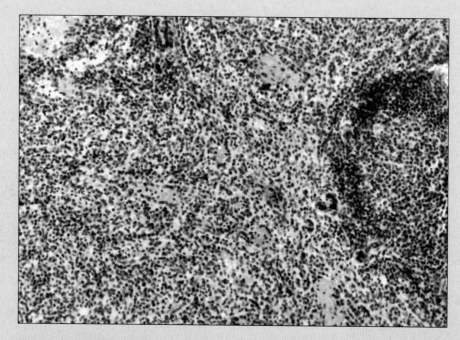

Figure 11-17 (50×): Spleen.

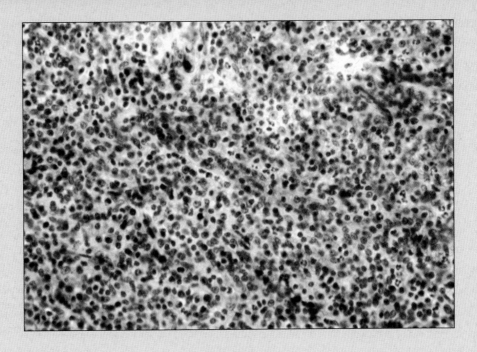

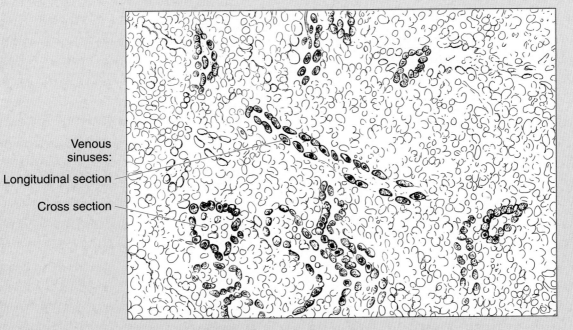

Venous
sinuses:

Longitudinal section

Cross section

Figure 11-18 (100×): Spleen.

Logic Tree

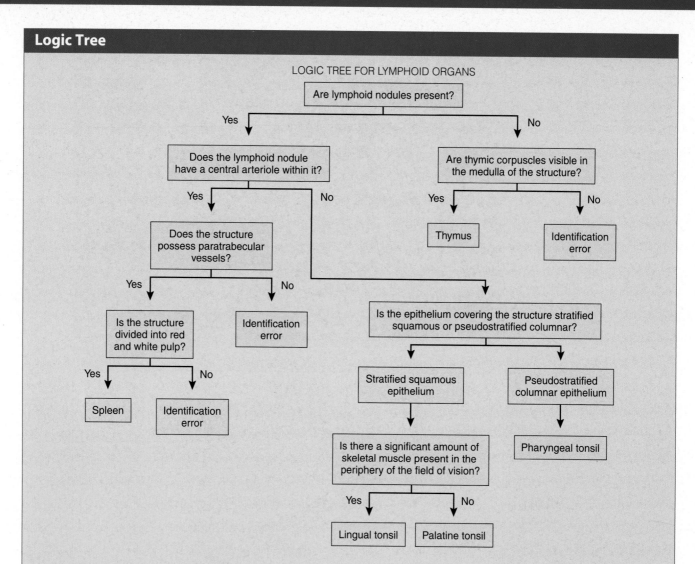

LOGIC TREE FOR LYMPHOID ORGANS

Chapter 12

URINARY SYSTEM

Chapter Objectives

This chapter will enable you to discuss and identify:

1. The various components of the kidney that may be distinguished with the light microscope

2. The components of the juxtaglomerular apparatus

3. The urinary bladder

4. The ureter

5. The female urethra and the spongy and prostatic segments of the male urethra

The functions of the urinary system are the formation of urine, fluid balance, the regulation of blood pressure and acid-base balance, and the formation of specific hormones. All of these functions are accomplished by a series of structures found within the kidneys. The remaining structures of the urinary system, termed the *extrarenal excretory structures,* are the ureters, urinary bladder, and urethra. These structures are responsible for the passage of urine from the kidney to the external environment.

Kidney

When you view the kidney at scanning power you will note the following histological characteristics:

- The kidney is covered by a fibroelastic capsule.

- The kidney is divided into a cortex and medulla.

- The border between renal cortex and renal medulla is marked by the presence of arcuate arteries and veins.

- Renal corpuscles and segments of the uriniferous tubules are found within the renal cortex.

- The medulla, although lacking renal corpuscles, does contain segments of the uriniferous tubules.

Renal Corpuscle

The capsule of the kidney, which is not visible in these photomicrographs, is composed of fibroelastic connective tissue. The kidney is subdivided into *cortex* and *medulla*, which contain the *uriniferous tubules* of the kidney. Each uriniferous tubule is composed of a nephron and a collecting duct. The nephron begins as a double-walled epithelial cup composed of the *glomerular capsule* (also termed *Bowman's space*) surrounding a tuft of capillaries termed the *glomerulus*. Both structures together form the renal (Malpighian) corpuscle.

The *glomerular capsule* (**Figures 12-1** and **12-2**) is composed of two continuous, simple squamous epithelial layers (see section on Simple Cuboidal and Simple Squamous Epithelia in Chapter 2). The inner *visceral layer* covers and closely invests the glomerular capillaries. The cells of this visceral layer are termed *podocytes*. In these photomicrographs, they are seen facing *capsular space* (also termed the *urinary* or *Bowman's space*).

Although it is not visible in **Figures 12-1** to **12-3**, the visceral layer of the renal corpuscle is continuous with the *parietal layer* at the vascular pole. The *parietal layer* (**Figure 12-3**) of the renal corpuscle is composed of a simple squamous epithelium resting on a thin basal lamina. A think layer of connective tissue surrounds it externally. The cells of the parietal layer are more uniform in thickness than those of the visceral layer.

In **Figure 12-3**, the *urinary pole* may be seen where the simple squamous epithelium of the parietal layer of the glomerular capsule is joined by the simple cuboidal epithelium of the proximal convoluted tubule.

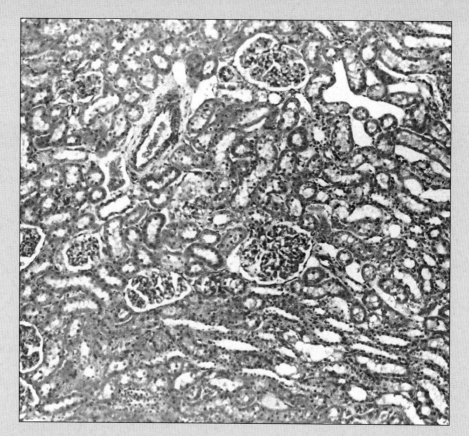

Figure 12-1 (25×): Renal corpuscle.

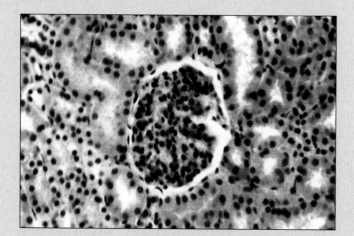

Figure 12-2 (100×): Renal corpuscle.

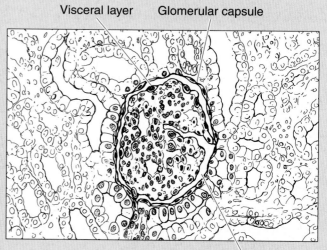

Visceral layer   Glomerular capsule

Capsular space

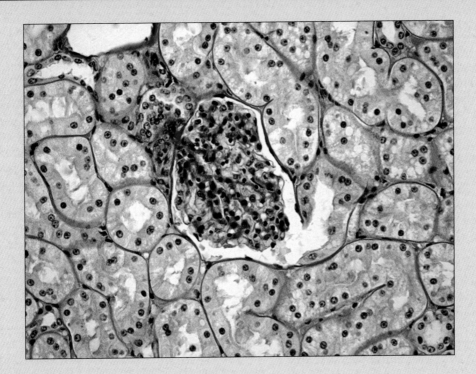

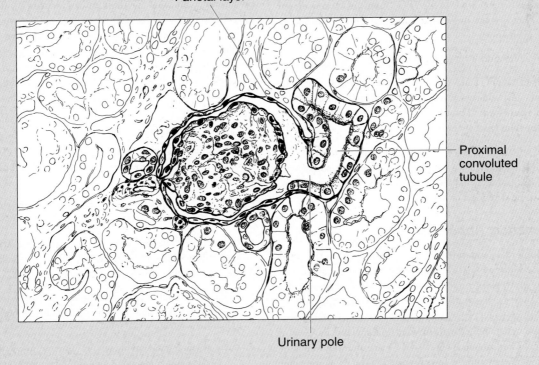

Parietal layer

Proximal
convoluted
tubule

Urinary pole

Figure 12-3 (250×): Renal corpuscle.

Proximal and Distal Convoluted Tubules

The tubular region of the nephron is composed of the proximal convoluted tubule, thick and thin segments of the nephron loop (loop of Henle), and the distal convoluted tubule. The *proximal convoluted tubule* (PCT) (Figure 12-4) is the longest and most convoluted segment of the nephron. Therefore the majority of the tubules found in the cortex will be PCT segments.

The PCT (Figure 12-4) is composed of simple cuboidal (or short columnar) epithelial cells. These cells possess a single, round nucleus in the basal portion of the cell, surrounded by granular, acidophilic cytoplasm. The lateral cellular boundaries of these cells are difficult to discern. Another characteristic of the PCT is a rounded, apical brush border that may be seen with high-dry or oil-immersion objectives. *Because of these overall characteristics, the PCT possess a small tubular lumen and a sparse distribution of nuclei around the circumference of the tubule; these are two important histological characteristics.*

The *distal convoluted tubule* (DCT) (Figure 12-4) is composed of a simple cuboidal epithelium. These cells also possess a granular cytoplasm but stain less intensely than those of the PCT. No brush border is visible on the apical portion of these cells. The overall size of the DCT cell is smaller, as evidenced by a larger tubular lumen. In addition, more nuclei are usually visible in the DCT.

The proximal convoluted tubule (PCT) and distal convoluted tubule (DCT) may be distinguished from each other by the following histological features:

- The PCT stains more intensely acidophilic.

- The cells of the PCT are cuboidal or short columnar epithelial cells, whereas those of the DCT are a shorter, cuboidal epithelium. Therefore the lumen of the PCT will be smaller than that of the DCT.

- The cells of the PCT have a prominent brush border on their apical surfaces. As a result of the close approximation of the brush borders of adjacent PCT cells, the lumen often appears to be occluded or star shaped.

Juxtaglomerular Apparatus

The juxtaglomerular apparatus (JGA) is found within the renal cortex of the kidney. It is located where the distal convoluted tubule comes into close proximity with the afferent glomerular arteriole at the vascular pole. The juxtaglomerular apparatus is composed of three cell types: macula densa cells, juxtaglomerular epithelioid cells, and extraglomerular mesangial cells.

The *macula densa cells* (Figure 12-5) are modified cells of the distal convoluted tubule (see Figure 12-4). They are taller and more rounded than other cells of the DCT and possess apical nuclei. Macula densa cells usually stain more acidophilic than the other DCT cells within the same tubule.

The second cell type, found where the afferent glomerular arteriole comes into close proximity to the macula densa, is termed the *juxtaglomerular epithelioid cell.* These cells are found within the wall of the afferent glomerular arteriole, where they form a collar within the tunica media. They are modified smooth muscle cells (see section on Smooth Muscle in Chapter 6) in that they are larger and more epithelioid in appearance than the other smooth muscle cells within the tunica media of the same arteriole.

The final cell type of the JGA is the extraglomerular mesangial cell (not visible on this photomicrograph). It is found between the afferent and efferent glomerular arterioles and therefore will be visible only in sections containing both arterioles. These cells are modified smooth muscle cells.

Collecting Duct (Collecting Tubule)

The *collecting ducts* (collecting tubules) may be found within the renal cortex; however, they are most numerous within the renal medulla (Figure 12-6). Cells of the collecting duct range in height from simple cuboidal to simple columnar (see section on Simple Columnar Epithelium in Chapter 2). The intercellular borders are quite distinct; the cells possess a rounded apical surface and stain less intensely than the other renal tubules.

The cells of the collecting duct may be distinguished from cells of the PCT (see section on the Proximal and Distal Convoluted Tubules in this chapter) and DCT by the following major histological features:

- Most segments of the collecting duct will be found within the medulla of the kidney, whereas proximal (PCT) and distal convoluted tubules (DCT) are most commonly seen within the renal cortex.

- Cells of the collecting duct tend to be smaller than those of the PCT or DCT.

- Cells of the collecting duct possess a rounded, apical surface, as do those of the PCT. However, cells of the collecting duct are considerably smaller than those of the PCT.

- Cells of the collecting duct stain less intensely than those of the PCT or DCT and lack the distinct brush border seen in cells of the PCT.

- Cells of the collecting duct have distinct intercellular boundaries that are not seen in the PCT or DCT.

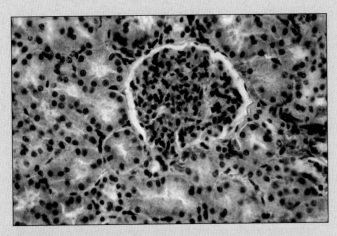

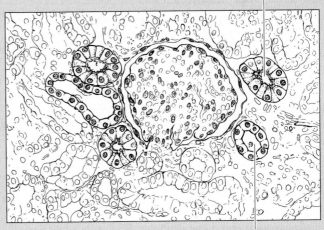

Proximal convoluted tubule

Distal convoluted tubule

Figure 12-4 (100×): Proximal and distal convoluted tubules.

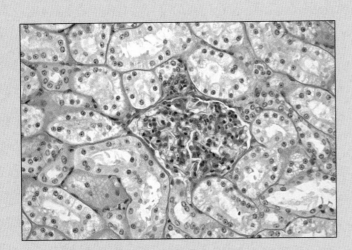

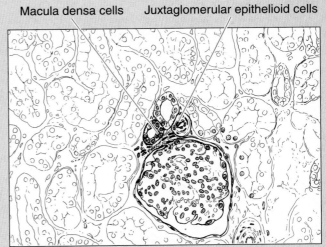

Macula densa cells   Juxtaglomerular epithelioid cells

Figure 12-5 (100×): Juxtaglomerular apparatus.

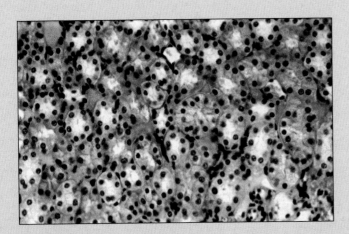

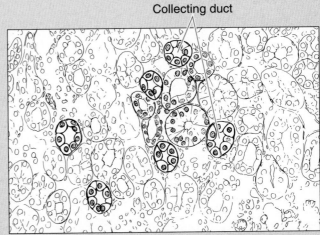

Collecting duct

Figure 12-6 (100×): Collecting duct.

Nephron Loop

Figure 12-7 is of the medulla of the kidney. The *thin limb of nephron loop* (loop of Henle) is lined by a simple squamous epithelium. The nuclei of these cells bulge into the lumen of the tubule and appear somewhat less flattened than the nuclei of the adjacent endothelial cells of the *vasa recta*.

Ureter

The ureter and renal pelvis, and its subdivisions, constitute the main excretory ducts of the kidney. The walls of the ureter are composed of three layers: an inner mucosa, a middle muscularis, and an outer adventitia. Because of the high content of elastic fibers within the wall of the ureter, the lumen is quite often star shaped.

The *mucosa* of the ureter (Figure 12-8) is lined by a transitional epithelium (see section on Transitional Epithelia in Chapter 2) sitting on a thin basal lamina that is not discernible with the light microscope. Diffuse lymphoid tissue (see section on Diffuse Lymphatic Tissue in Chapter 11) may be present within the *lamina propria*.

The *muscularis* in the upper two thirds of the ureter is composed of two layers of smooth muscle—an *inner longitudinal* and *outer circular layer*. In the inferior one third of the ureter, an additional layer might be present, represented by a discontinuous outer longitudinal layer of smooth muscle.

The *adventitia* is composed of areolar connective tissue with numerous blood vessels. It may not be present in all sections.

Urinary Bladder

Urinary Bladder (Relaxed)

The wall of the urinary bladder is quite similar to that of the ureter, except for the increased thickness of the muscularis.

The *mucosa* of the urinary bladder (Figures 12-9 and 2-15) is composed of a transitional epithelium (see Figure 2-15) resting on a thin basal lamina and a lamina propria. The mucosa may be thrown into folds or may be comparatively smooth, depending on the state of stretch of the organ at the time of fixation.

The muscularis is rather thick, possessing three layers of smooth muscle: inner and outer longitudinal layers and a middle circular layer. This is a major histological feature of the urinary bladder. The fiber bundles are arranged in anastomosing bundles with connective tissue between the layers.

The adventitia of the lower bladder (if visible in your section) is identical to that of the ureter, whereas that of the upper two thirds possesses an outer serosa composed of a mesothelium and loose connective tissue.

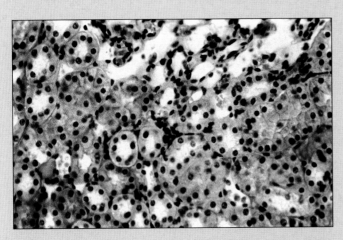

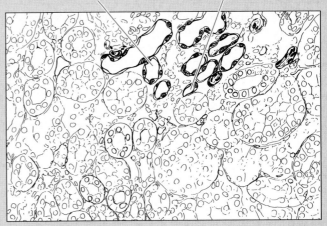

Thin segment of nephron loop   Vasa recta

Figure 12-7 (100×): Thin segment of the nephron loop (of Henle).

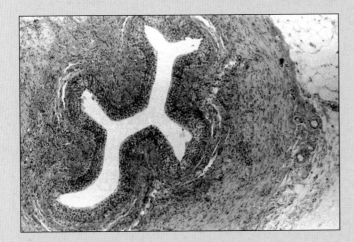

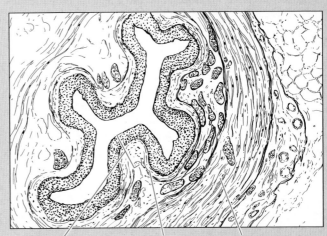

Mucosa   Lamina propria   Muscularis

Figure 12-8 (25×): Ureter (cross section).

Muscularis   Mucosa

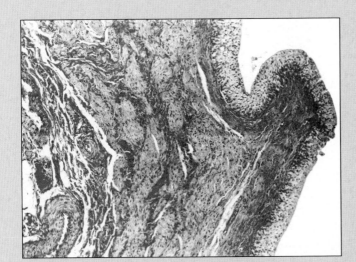

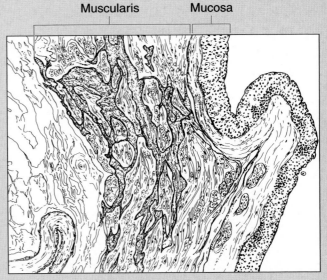

Figure 12-9 (25×): Urinary bladder (relaxed).

Urinary Bladder (Distended)

In the distended urinary bladder, the transitional epithelium may be reduced to as few as three layers of epithelial cells. Note that the superficial layer of cells in Figure 12-10 is squamosal in shape, whereas the deeper epithelial cells are quite variable in shape. Compare Figures 12-10 and 2-15 to note the differences between the transitional epithelium of a relaxed bladder and that of a distended bladder. *Because the most superficial layers of epithelial cells in a distended urinary bladder do not possess the "typical" transitional epithelium shape (described as dome shaped, balloon shaped, broadly cuboidal, or somewhat flattened) the identification of a distended urinary bladder must be based on the three layers of smooth muscle found within the muscularis of the bladder.*

Urethra

Male

Prostatic Urethra

The male urethra is subdivided into three regions: prostatic urethra, intermediate part of the urethra (membranous urethra), and spongy urethra. Figure 12-11 is a photomicrograph of the prostatic urethra.

The *mucosa* of the prostatic urethra possesses a transitional epithelium resting on a lamina propria that consists of fibroelastic connective tissue with prominent venous sinuses. The lumen of the prostatic urethra is irregular in shape because of the folding of the mucosa.

Throughout the entire length of the male urethra, numerous outfoldings of the mucosa may be seen. These are the *urethral glands* (glands of Littre). In the prostatic urethra, these branched, tubular glands extend for variable distances into the stroma of the prostate gland.

The muscularis (which is not clearly visible on this photomicrograph) consists of two indistinguishable layers: an inner longitudinal and an outer circular layer of smooth muscle. The adventitia (also not visible) is composed of fibroelastic areolar connective tissue.

Although the histology of the prostate is not discussed until Chapter 14, note its general histological organization, because the presence or absence of the prostate will aid you in your identification of male and female urethra specimens.

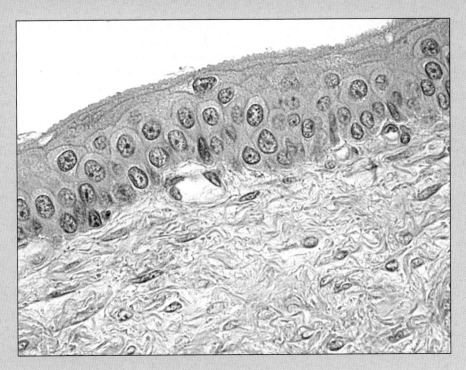

Figure 12-10 (40×): Urinary bladder (distended).

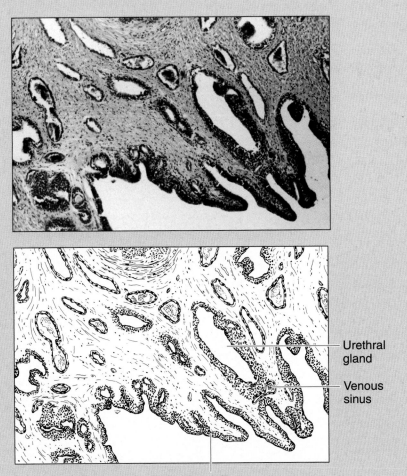

Urethral gland

Venous sinus

Epithelium of mucosa

Figure 12-11 (25×): Male prostatic urethra.

Penis/Spongy Urethra

Figure 12-12 is a line drawing of a human penis. The spongy urethra is found within the inferior, medial erectile body of the penis. *The presence of erectile bodies is a major histological feature of the spongy urethra.*

This section is from a human penis. Other slides used for specimens of the spongy urethra may have been obtained from animals possessing an os penis, identified by the presence of bone within the section.

The epithelium of the *mucosa* (Figure 12-13) within the spongy urethra varies from location to location, from stratified columnar to pseudostratified columnar (see sections on Stratified Columnar Epithelium and Pseudostratified Columnar Epithelium in Chapter 2). Smooth muscle fibers may be found within the mucosa. A lamina propria of fibroelastic connective tissue is found immediately deep to the epithelium. The mucosa of the spongy urethra possesses urethral glands (glands of Littre; not visible on this section), which may extend deep into the stroma and penetrate into the corpus spongiosum.

Although the histology of the penis is not discussed until Chapter 14, note its general histological organization. The presence or absence of the penis will aid you in your identification of male and female urethra specimens.

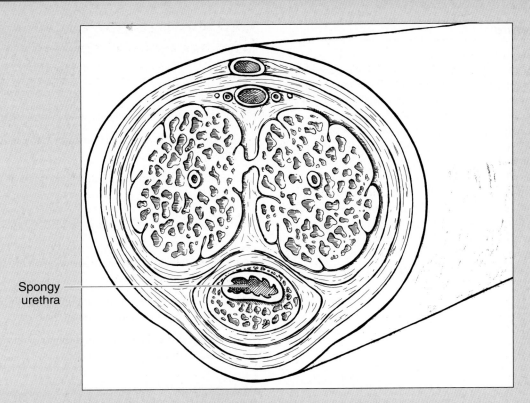

Figure 12-12 Line drawing of a cross section of a human penis.

Spongy
urethra

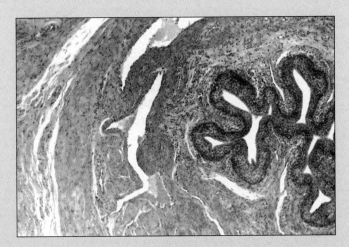

Figure 12-13 (25×): Human penis (cross section).

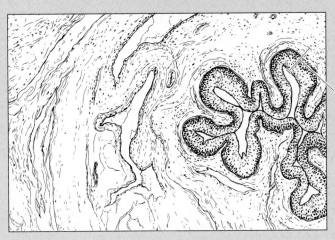

Mucosa

Female Urethra

The epithelium of the *mucosa* (Figures 12-14 and 12-15) will vary considerably from individual to individual. Near the bladder it is usually transitional; the remainder of the female urethra may be lined with stratified squamous, stratified columnar epithelium or pseudostratified columnar epithelium. The mucosa is thrown into *longitudinal folds*, and *urethral glands* are also visible in Figure 12-15. *There are fewer urethral glands in the female urethra than in the male urethra; this is a major histological feature of this specimen.* The stroma of the mucosa is rich in elastic fibers, owing to the longitudinal folding of the female urethra.

The *muscularis* (see Figure 12-14) is rather indefinite yet contains both longitudinal and circular layers of smooth muscle. An outer layer of skeletal muscle (not visible on this photomicrograph) may be present if your section was taken at the site of the voluntary sphincter. A definite adventitia is absent.

Commonly Misidentified Tissues

Ureter and Relaxed Urinary Bladder

Ureter (Review **Figure 12-8** in section on the Ureter)

1. Mucosa is folded, usually resulting in a star-shaped lumen.

2. Epithelium of the mucosa is uniform in thickness around the entire lumen.

3. Muscularis is composed of either two layers of smooth muscle.

Urinary Bladder (Review **Figure 12-9** in section on the Urinary Bladder [Relaxed])

1. Mucosal folding is variable, depending on the state of organ distension at fixation.

2. Epithelium of the mucosa is not uniform in thickness, owing to the variable distention of the organ.

3. Although it may be difficult to distinguish, the muscularis is always composed of three layers.

Commonly Misidentified Tissues

Male and Female Urethra

Male Urethra (Prostatic or Spongy) (Review **Figure 12-12** in section on the Penis/Spongy Urethra)

1. Presence of prostate gland (with its numerous outpocketings surrounding prostatic urethra) or penile tissue surrounding urethra

2. Urethral glands very prominent. Muscularis absent in two of three regions (being present only in the intermediate part of the urethra)

Female Urethra (Review **Figures 12-14** and **12-15** in section on the Female Urethra)

1. Prostate gland or penile erectile tissue absent

2. Voluntary sphincter and corresponding outer layer of skeletal muscle usually present

3. Urethral glands present but in a reduced number

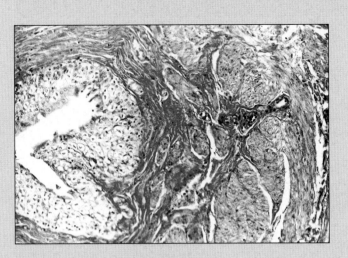

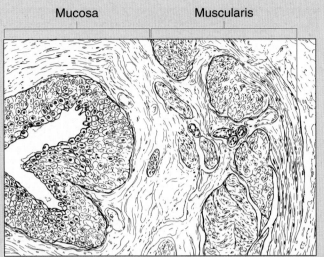

Mucosa   Muscularis

Figure 12-14 (25×): Female urethra.

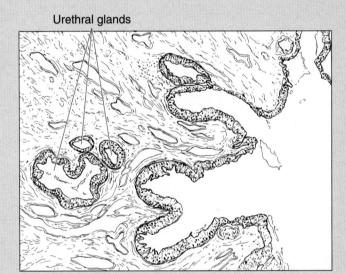

Urethral glands

Figure 12-15 (50×): Female urethra.

Logic Tree

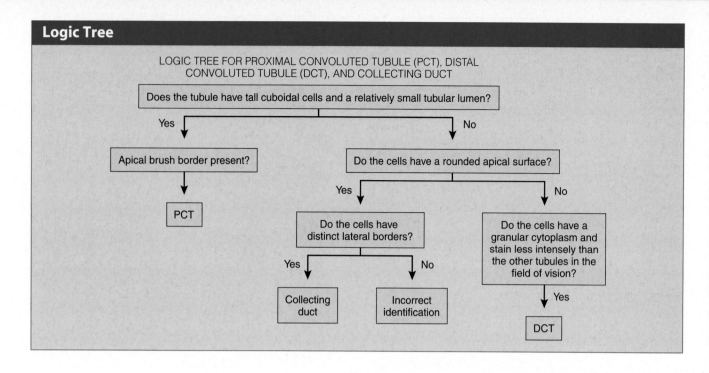

LOGIC TREE FOR PROXIMAL CONVOLUTED TUBULE (PCT), DISTAL
CONVOLUTED TUBULE (DCT), AND COLLECTING DUCT

Does the tubule have tall cuboidal cells and a relatively small tubular lumen?

Yes — Apical brush border present? → PCT

No — Do the cells have a rounded apical surface?

Yes — Do the cells have distinct lateral borders?
- Yes → Collecting duct
- No → Incorrect identification

No — Do the cells have a granular cytoplasm and stain less intensely than the other tubules in the field of vision?
- Yes → DCT

Logic Tree

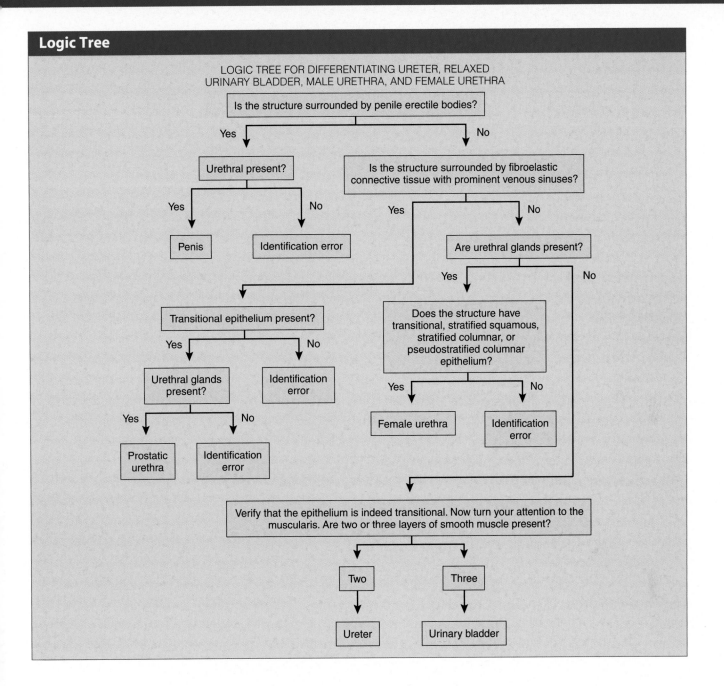

LOGIC TREE FOR DIFFERENTIATING URETER, RELAXED URINARY BLADDER, MALE URETHRA, AND FEMALE URETHRA

Chapter 13

ENDOCRINE SYSTEM

Chapter Objectives

This chapter will enable you to identify the:

1. Cell types of the adenohypophysis (anterior pituitary or pars distalis) and neurohypophysis (posterior pituitary or pars nervosa)

2. Components and cell types of the thyroid and parathyroid glands

3. Regions and cell types of the suprarenal cortex and suprarenal medulla

4. Pancreatic islets (Islets of Langerhans) within the pancreas

5. Components and cell types of the pineal gland

Characteristics of Endocrine Glands

An endocrine gland is defined as a ductless gland that releases its secretions directly onto the surface of the cell or directly into the lymphoid system, interstitial fluids, or bloodstream. Whether the endocrine gland constitutes only a small portion of the gland (as in the pancreas) or makes up the majority of the gland, all endocrine glands share several characteristics:

- The cells secreting the hormones possess either neural, epithelial, or epithelioid characteristics.

- All endocrine glands are richly vascularized.

- The glands either lack ducts or the ducts do not communicate with the endocrine portion of the organ.

Endocrine glands produce three major types of hormones: (1) steroids, (2) proteins or polypeptides, and (3) neurotransmitter substances. The ultrastructure of these cells will mirror the type of hormone produced. Although the ultrastructure of endocrine cells is not visible with the light microscope, it will affect the histological characteristics of the cells.

Steroid hormones are produced by endocrine cells that:

- Have an abundant smooth endoplasmic reticulum (SER), thereby causing the cytoplasm of the cells to stain acidophilically

- Have numerous mitochondria with tubular cristae, again causing the cytoplasm to stain acidophilically

- Contain lipid droplets within the cytoplasm. These droplets are dissolved during the fixation process, thereby making the cytoplasm of the cells stain lightly.

Protein and polypeptide hormones are produced by endocrine cells that:

- Have an abundant rough endoplasmic reticulum (RER) and Golgi apparatus. If these cells are actively synthesizing hormones, the cytoplasm will stain predominantly basophilic, owing to the large amounts of tRNA, mRNA, and ribosomal RNA within the cytoplasm.

- Frequently possess membrane-bound secretory granules, thereby giving the cytoplasm a slightly granular appearance.

Neurotransmitter substances are produced by endocrine cells that:

- Are derived from embryonic central nervous system tissues and therefore typically retain many of the histological characteristics seen in nervous tissue.

Pituitary Gland (Hypophysis)

The pituitary gland (hypophysis) is divided into an adenohypophysis (anterior lobe) and the neurohypophysis (posterior lobe). The adenohypophysis is further subdivided into the pars distalis (also termed the *pars anterior*), pars intermedia, and pars tuberalis, and the neurohypophysis is subdivided into the infundibulum and the neural lobe (posterior lobe). We will confine our histological examination of the pituitary gland to the pars distalis of the adenohypophysis and the neural lobe of the neurohypophysis.

Pars Distalis of the Adenohypophysis

The pars distalis (anterior lobe) of the adenohypophysis of the pituitary gland possesses a parenchyma of anastomosing cords of cells separated from sinusoidal capillaries by a small amount of irregular connective tissue (Figures 13-1 and 13-2). The parenchymal cells of the adenohypophysis are separated into two categories: *chromophils* and *chromophobes* (Figure 13-2). The granules within the cytoplasm of chromophils will stain with either eosin or hematoxylin, whereas those within chromophobes will not react with either stain or will do so very poorly.

Chromophils are further subdivided into *acidophils* (alpha cells) and *basophils* (beta cells) (Figure 13-2). Cytoplasmic granules determine the staining properties of the chromophils. Eosin will stain the granules of the acidophils; the granules of the basophils will stain poorly, or not at all, with hematoxylin. They will, however, stain quite well with aniline blue or Masson's trichrome stains. Basophils on these photomicrographs stain lightly basophilic.

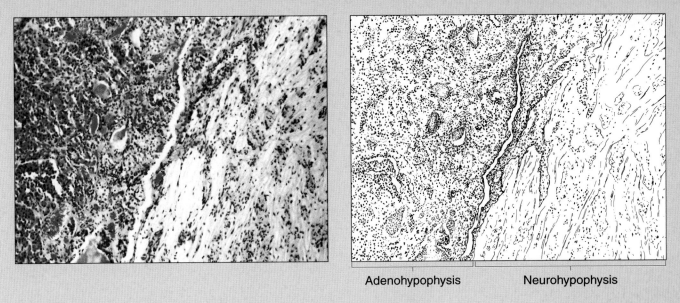

Adenohypophysis   Neurohypophysis

Figure 13-1 (25×): Pars distalis of the adenohypophysis (anterior lobe) of the pituitary.

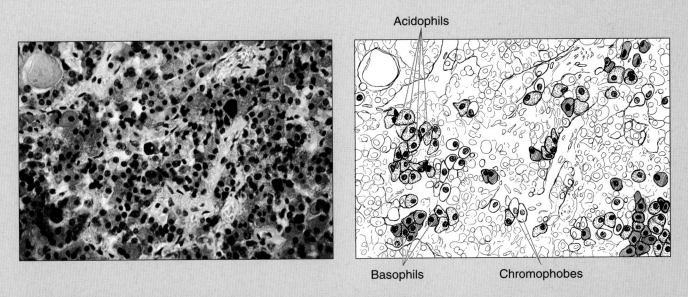

Acidophils

Basophils   Chromophobes

Figure 13-2 (100×): Pars distalis of the adenohypophysis (anterior lobe) of the pituitary.

Neural Lobe of the Neurohypophysis

The *neural lobe* (pars nervosa) contains unmyelinated axons from the hypothalamo-hypophysial tract, blood vasculature, and *pituicytes*. In routine hematoxylin and eosin sections (Figure 13-3), the neural lobe is quite bland in that the individual axons cannot be easily distinguished, and the pituicytes resemble neuroglial cells in many ways (see sections on the Spinal Cord and Cerebral Cortex in Chapter 7).

Pituicytes (Figures 13-3 and 13-4) are small cells with ramifying processes that cannot be observed with the light micro-scope. Their nuclei are either round or oval and possess fine chromatin. In routine histological preparations, the cytoplasm of these cells is faintly visible.

Within the neural lobe, *neurosecretory bodies* (also termed *Herring Bodies*) may also be seen (Figure 13-4). These are large accumulations of neurosecretory material and degradative products within individual axons and nerve endings. Neurosecretory bodies appear as brown or reddish-brown granules between the pituicytes of the posterior pituitary.

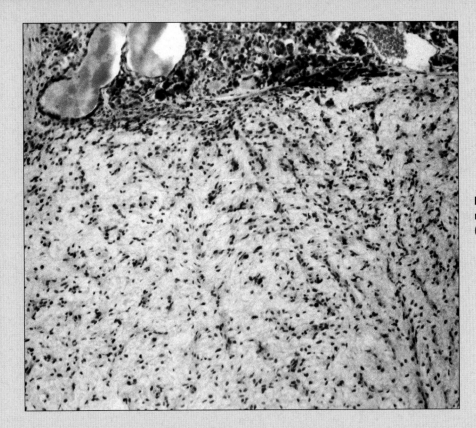

Figure 13-3 (25×): Neural lobe (pars nervosa) of the neurohypophysis (posterior lobe) of the pituitary.

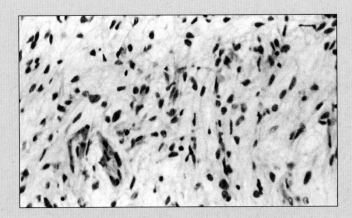

Figure 13-4 (100×): Neural lobe (pars nervosa) of the neurohypophysis (posterior lobe) of the pituitary.

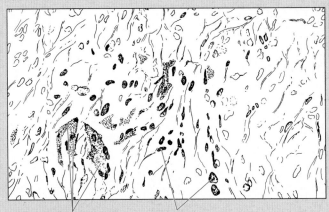

Neurosecretory bodies   Pituicytes

Thyroid and Parathyroid Glands

Thyroid Gland

A true connective tissue capsule composed of fibroelastic connective tissue surrounds the thyroid gland (Figure 13-5). Delicate trabeculae and septa (which are not visible on this photomicrograph) radiate inward from the capsule.

The structural unit of the thyroid, the *follicle*, has an irregular spherical shape (Figures 13-5 and 13-6). The follicle contains an internal *follicular cavity* filled with a gel-like material termed *colloid*. The *T thyrocytes* of the follicular epithelium are simple cuboidal epithelial cells (see section on Simple Cuboidal Epithelia in Chapter 2), and their height will vary slightly, depending on their synthetic activity.

In this photomicrograph, the intercellular boundaries between the T thyrocytes are distinct. The cells possess a rounded nucleus within a lightly basophilic cytoplasm (Figure 13-6). The staining properties of the follicular epithelium will range from lightly basophilic for inactive squamous or cuboidal cells to deeply basophilic for cuboidal to columnar follicular epithelium with a high synthetic activity. The apical ends of the cells possess microvilli that may be visible under oil immersion.

C *thyrocytes* (parafollicular cells, "C" cells, clear cells, or calcitonin cells) should be visible on your section (Figure 13-6). These cells may be found either singly or in groups and may be found in the wall of the follicle or in the interfollicular space. Generally, they are larger than the T thyrocytes and stain very lightly. They are relatively sparse in humans. Why?

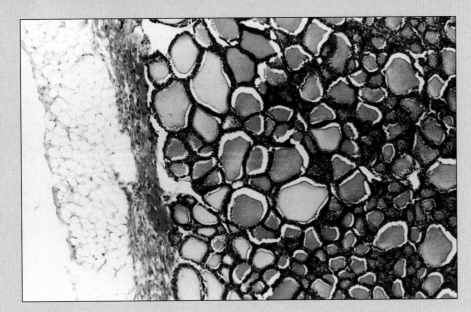

Figure 13-5 (25×): Thyroid gland.

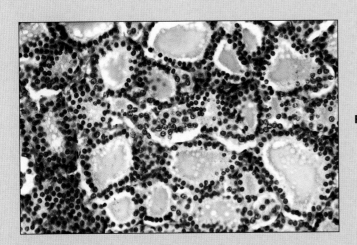

Figure 13-6 (100×): Thyroid gland.

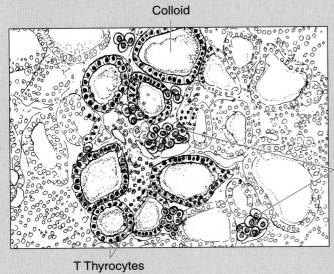

Colloid

C Thyrocytes

T Thyrocytes

Parathyroid Gland

The parathyroid gland possesses a delicate connective tissue *capsule* with slight septa radiating inward. These septa separate the parenchyma into anastomosing cords, a feature that becomes more obvious in the adult because of the increase amount of adipose tissue within the gland (Figure 13-7) (see section on White [unilocular] Adipose Tissue in Chapter 3).

The parenchyma of the parathyroid gland is composed of three cell types: *parathyroid cells* (also called *chief cells* or *principle cells*), *oxyphil cells*, and transition cells (Figure 13-8).

Parathyroid cells are constant in number and occurrence. They are polyhedral in shape, possess sparse cytoplasm, and have a rounded nucleus with loosely arranged chromatin. They possess a pale, slightly eosinophilic cytoplasm.

Oxyphil cells do not appear until after the first decade of life and are not abundant until puberty. They may be found scattered throughout the gland and occur either singly or in clumps. They are larger than parathyroid cells, with smaller yet darker-staining nuclei. The cytoplasm stains deeply with eosin.

Transitional cells possess cytological characteristics intermediate between those of the parathyroid and oxyphil cells and cannot be easily distinguished with the light microscope.

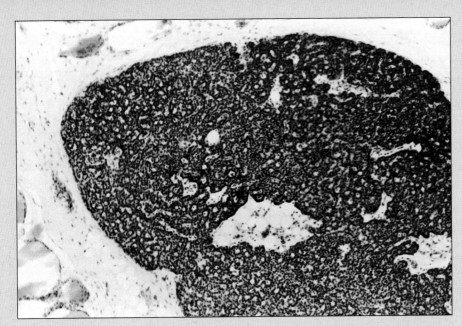

Figure 13-7 (25×): Parathyroid gland.

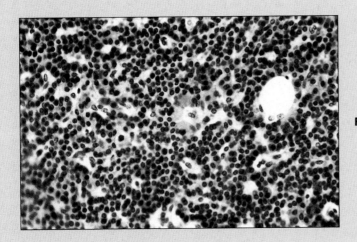

Figure 13-8 (100×): Parathyroid gland.

Parathyroid cell

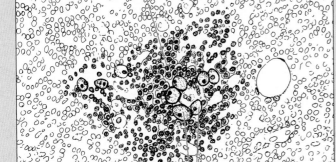

Oxyphil cells

Suprarenal (Adrenal) Gland

Suprarenal Cortex

The suprarenal glands (Figure 13-9) (also called the *adrenal glands*) are actually composite glands, being composed of a *cortex* and a *medulla*, each of which has a different embryonic origin and produces different secretions. The cortex originates from mesodermal cells of the nephrogenic ridge and produces steroids; the medulla has its embryonic origin in the neural crest and produces epinephrine and norepinephrine. Therefore the appearance and staining qualities of these two sections will be quite different.

The suprarenal gland is covered with a thick *capsule*, composed chiefly of collagen (Figure 13-9). Delicate trabeculae extend inward from the capsule. The arrangement into *cortex* and *medulla* is not uniform in human suprarenal glands but is quite distinct in the suprarenal glands of many animals.

Figure 13-10 shows the outer portion of the suprarenal cortex, which is divided into three zones. The outermost zone is relatively thin and is termed the *zona glomerulosa;* the cells of this zone are arranged into ovoid groups. Their cytoplasm contains lipid droplets that are dissolved during the fixation process, and therefore they may appear as vacuoles. The nuclei stain darkly.

The *zona fasciculata* is the largest of the three zones, and the cells are arranged into long, parallel cords that are one to two cells thick and course perpendicular to the capsule. The cells are cuboidal or polyhedral in shape and may possess two nuclei. Because of a high concentration of lipid droplets within the cytoplasm, these cells stain lightly and have a vacuolated (spongy) appearance. These cells are sometimes referred to as *spongiocytes*.

The innermost zone is the *zona reticularis* and is composed of a network of cords (Figure 13-11). These cells are considerably smaller than those of the zona fasciculata, stain more acidophilic (Figure 13-10), and frequently have nuclei that stain more deeply. Lipofuscin granules may be evident within the cytoplasm of these cells when viewed with the oil-immersion lens.

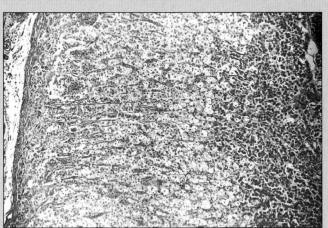

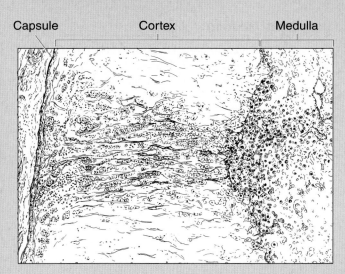

Capsule   Cortex   Medulla

Figure 13-9 (25×): Suprarenal gland.

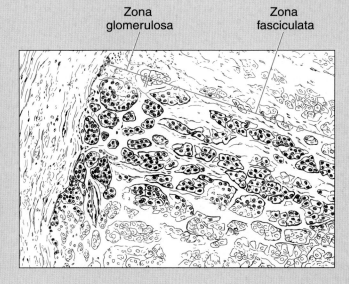

Zona glomerulosa   Zona fasciculata

Figure 13-10 (50×): Suprarenal gland.

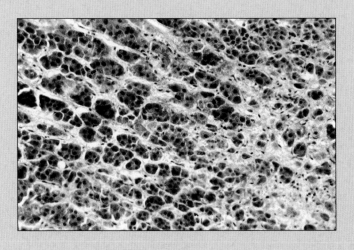

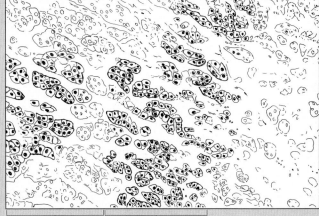

Zona fasciculata   Zona reticularis

Figure 13-11 (50×): Suprarenal gland.

Suprarenal Medulla

The cells of the medulla are arranged into anastomosing cords and are termed *chromaffin cells* (Figure 13-12). They are polygonal to columnar in shape and contain fine cytoplasmic granules that may be seen when viewed with the oil-immersion lens.

Endocrine Pancreas/Pancreatic Islets

The pancreas is a composite gland with both exocrine and endocrine functions. The endocrine pancreas is composed of the *pancreatic islets* (also termed *Islets of Langerhans*). These cells are in the form of a spherical mass of pale staining cells arranged into irregularly anastomosing cords (Figure 13-13). Numerous capillaries (see section on Capillaries in Chapter 8) are found between the cells.

Chromaffin cells

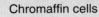

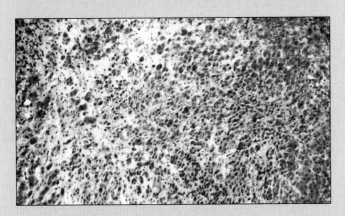

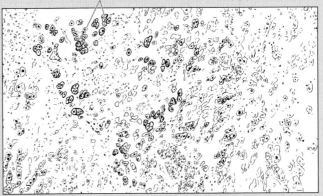

Figure 13-12 (50×): Suprarenal gland.

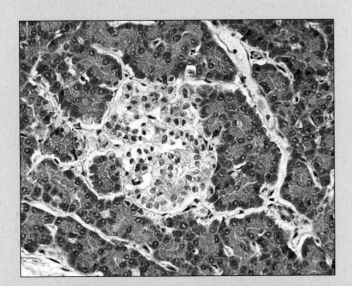

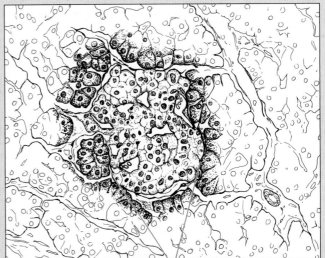

Pancreatic islet

Figure 13-13 (100×): Pancreatic islet (Islet of Langerhans) of the pancreas.

Pineal Gland

The pineal gland (pineal body) is an endocrine or neuroendocrine gland attached to the roof of the diencephalon at the posterior wall of the third ventricle, near the center of the brain. The *pia mater* may be seen on the right side of **Figure 13-14**. *Acervulus* (also termed *corpora arenacea* or *brain sand*), *which is a major identification feature of the pineal gland*, may be seen in this photomicrograph. The number of corpora arenacea within the pineal gland increases with age. These structures appear to be calcium phosphate and calcium carbonate precipitates found on carrier proteins that have been released by exocytosis.

The pineal gland contains two cell types: *pinealocytes* and *astrocytes of the pineal gland* (also termed *interstitial glial cells*) **(Figure 13-15)**. *Pinealocytes* are arranged into cords or clumps that extend deep into the gland. They have a prominent nucleus that often appears infolded. One or two prominent nucleoli may be evident within the nucleus.

Astrocytes of the pineal gland make up approximately 5% of the cells within the pineal gland. These cells have cytological and staining characteristics similar to other glial cells within the central nervous system.

Commonly Misidentified Tissues

Parathyroid, Thymus, Lymph Node, and Spleen

Although the various endocrine glands are easy to differentiate, you may encounter difficulty distinguishing between the parathyroid gland and various glands of the lymphoid system. Therefore, keep the following histological characteristics in mind in order to differentiate between these organs.

Parathyroid Gland (Review **Figures 13-7** and **13-8** in section on the Parathyroid Gland)

1. Differential staining of the cells within the gland, owing to the presence of oxyphil and parathyroid cells

2. Cells arranged into cords

3. Prominent capillary bed without sinuses

4. Very thin capsule

Thymus Gland (Review **Figures 11-10** to **11-13** in section on the Thymus in Chapter 11)

1. Arrangement into cortex and medulla

2. Thymic (Hassal's) corpuscles present within the medulla

3. Cells within gland possess uniform staining qualities.

4. Very thin capsule

Lymph Node (Review **Figures 11-6** to **11-9** in section on Lymph Nodes in Chapter 11)

1. Lymphoid nodules with germinal centers are present.

2. Medullary sinuses are prominent.

3. Cells of the cortex are not arranged into cords.

4. Capsule is thicker than that of endocrine glands but thinner than that of spleen.

5. There are definitive subcapsular and paratrabecular spaces.

Spleen (Review **Figures 11-14** to **11-18** in section on the Spleen in Chapter 11)

1. Lymphoid nodules with germinal centers present

2. Central arteries present within germinal centers

3. Capsule thicker than that of lymph node

4. Differentiation into red and white pulp

5. No cortex or medulla

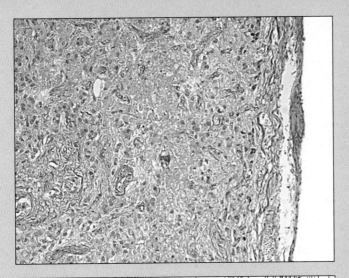

Figure 13-14 (35×): Pineal gland.

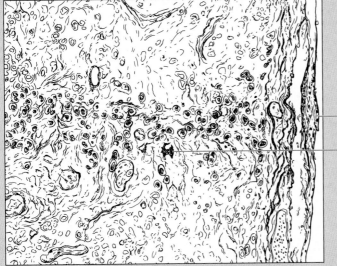

— Pia mater

— Acervulus
(Brain sand)

Astrocyte of pineal gland   Pinealocytes

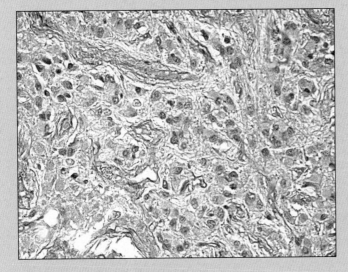

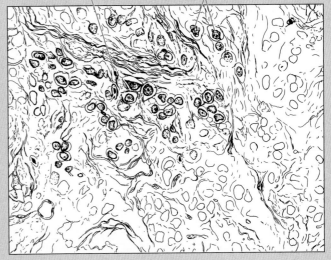

Figure 13-15 (70×): Pineal gland.

MALE REPRODUCTIVE SYSTEM

Components of the Male Reproductive System and Their Functions

The male reproductive system is responsible for the production of male sex hormones and the formation and delivery of spermatozoa, in the form of semen, to the female reproductive system. The organs responsible for these functions are:

- Testis (spermatogenesis and production of male sex hormones)

- Duct system (spermatogenesis and the delivery of semen to the urethra)

- Accessory glands (production of fluid components of semen)

Testis

Seminiferous Tubules

The testis is covered externally on its anterior and lateral aspects by a mesothelial layer of simple squamous epithelium termed the *tunica vaginalis.* (Not visible in these photomicrographs.) Deep to the tunica vaginalis you will find the tough connective tissue capsule of the testis, the *tunica albuginea* (Figure 14-1).

The tunica albuginea is composed of coarse, interweaving, collagenous fibers. The inner portion of the capsule is termed the *vascular layer of the testis* (also termed the *tunica vasculosa*), which is composed of a looser, highly vascularized layer of con-

nective tissue. Extensions of the vascular layer extend inward as *connective tissue septa*, which divide the testis into numerous lobules.

Deep to the vascular layer of the testis you will find the *seminiferous tubules* (Figure 14-1). These tubules are composed of a complex, stratified epithelium (see section on Stratified Epithelia in Chapter 2) resting on a thick, basal lamina and alternating layers of collagen fibers and flattened cells termed *myoid cells.* Peripheral to the myoid cells may also be a layer of fibroblasts and fibrocytes.

The epithelium of the seminiferous tubules is composed of *nurse cells* (also termed *Sertoli cells*) and *spermatogenic cells* (Figure 14-2). Nurse cells are the only cells that extend from the basal lamina to the tubular lumen; they form the major structural component of the seminiferous tubules. However, because of their staining characteristics it is difficult, if not impossible, to discern the apical portion of a nurse cell with the light microscope. Therefore nurse cells do not appear to extend from the basal lamina to the tubular lumen in a typical hematoxylin and eosin (H & E) preparation.

Nurse cells are slender and elongated, with irregular lateral outlines that are not visible with the light microscope. The cytoplasm of these cells often exhibits faint longitudinal striations. The distinctive nucleus is ovoid or somewhat triangular in shape, clearly outlined, and pale staining, with fine, sparse chromatin. One or more prominent nucleoli are often seen within the nucleus of a nurse cell, and the position of the nucleus may vary from cell to cell.

Spermatogenesis is the process by which sperm are produced by the testis. During this process, spermatogonial cells undergo a series of developmental changes and cellular mitotic and meiotic divisions. Only two stages of spermatogenesis will be addressed in this photomicrograph.

Within the seminiferous tubules of **Figure 14-2** you should be able to identify *late spermatids,* which are usually located closest to the tubular lumen. Late spermatids have prominent tails that extend into the lumen and nuclei that are small and bullet shaped. In many H & E preparations only the nucleus is visible.

Near the basal lamina of the seminiferous tubules of **Figure 14-2** you should be able to identify *primary spermatocytes.* These spherical cells demonstrate a significant clumping of the chromatin.

Not every seminiferous tubule will contain spermatogenic cells in the same state of differentiation. If you wish to identify the various stages of spermatogenesis, you may have to use numerous fields of vision to see them. Other stages that may be found in H & E preparations (but are not labeled on this photomicrograph) would include early spermatids, secondary spermatocytes, and Type A and Type B spermatogonia.

Located within the stroma and between the seminiferous tubules in **Figure 14-3** are the *interstitial endocrine cells* (interstitial cells of Leydig). These cells, which usually occur in groups, are large and ovoid and possess a large, eccentrically located nucleus. The cytoplasm is granular and fairly dense near the nucleus, whereas the peripheral cytoplasm is vesicular and vacuolated. These cells will stain lightly acidophilic in H & E preparations because of the large number of cytoplasmic lipid droplets.

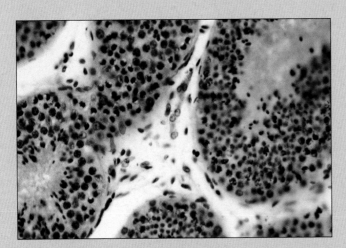

Figure 14-1 (25×): Testis.

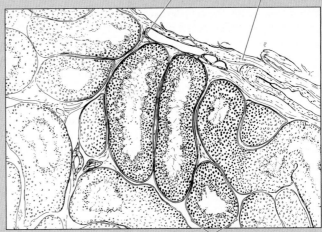

Septa   Tunica albuginea

Seminiferous
tubule

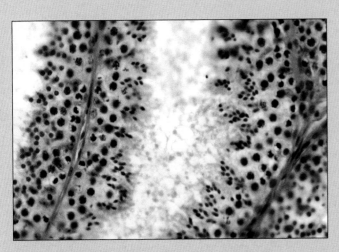

Figure 14-2 (100×): Testis.

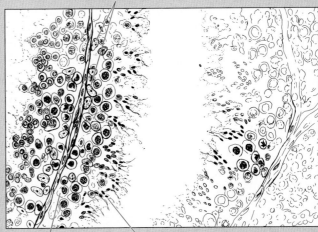

Nurse cells

Primary
spermatocyte   Late spermatid

Interstitial endocrine cells

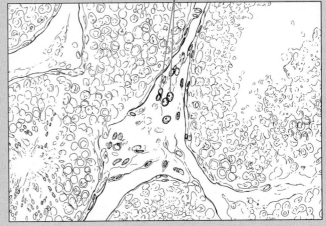

Figure 14-3 (100×): Interstitial cells (of Leydig).

Rete Testis

When looking for the rete testis on a slide it is important to orientate yourself first at low power. Follow the tunica albuginea around the periphery of the section until you locate the posterior surface of the testis, where the tunica albuginea thickens and invaginates. This invagination is termed the *mediastinum* of the testis; it is the location of the rete testis (Figure 14-4).

The *rete testis* is composed of wide, anastomosing channels lined with simple cuboidal epithelium (see section on Simple Cuboidal Epithelia in Chapter 2). The nuclei of the rete stain deeply, and the lateral borders of the cells are well defined under higher magnifications. No definite lamina propria is seen deep to the epithelium because of the connective tissue of the surrounding mediastinum.

Efferent Ductules and Epididymis

Sperm are transported from the rete testis to the epididymis via the efferent ductules. The *efferent ductules* (Figure 14-5) possess an epithelium composed of high columnar cells alternating with low columnar cells, *thereby giving the lumen a scalloped appearance*. This epithelium is pseudostratified columnar (see section on Pseudostratified Epithelia in Chapter 2), but it does not resemble that of the respiratory system (see section on the Trachea in Chapter 10). Some of the tall cells will possess cilia, and the epithelium rests on a distinct basal lamina. Deep to the lamina propria will be smooth muscle (see section on Smooth Muscle in Chapter 6) and a rich capillary network (see section on Capillaries in Chapter 8).

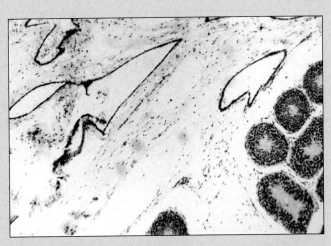

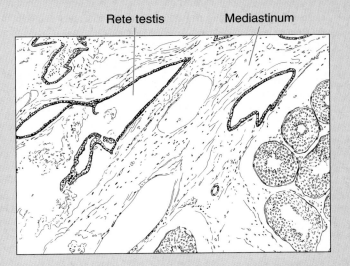

Rete testis Mediastinum

Figure 14-4 (25×): Rete testis.

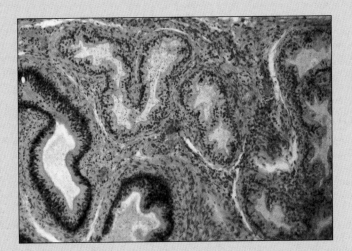

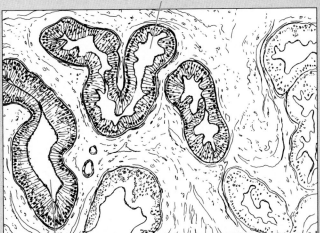

Ductule efferentes

Epididymus

Figure 14-5 (25×): Efferent ductules.

The epididymis is the site of sperm maturation and is subdivided into three regions: head, body, and tail. In contrast to the efferent ductules, the *epididymis* (Figure 14-6) *presents smooth internal and external contours*. The epithelium is pseudostratified columnar and is composed of *tall, columnar principal cells* and intermittent *basal cells*. The tall columnar cells are uniform in height and have numerous long, branching microvilli termed *stereocilia*.

Penis

Before studying the histology of the penis, review its gross anatomy by reexamining the structures seen in Figure 14-7. Note that the penis is composed of three cylindrical bodies:

- Two corpora cavernosa located dorsally

- One corpus spongiosum located inferiorly and seen to contain the spongy urethra

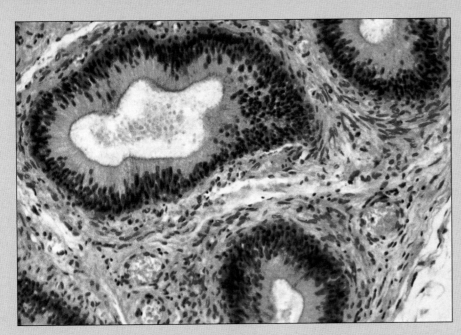

Figure 14-6 (50×): Epididymis.

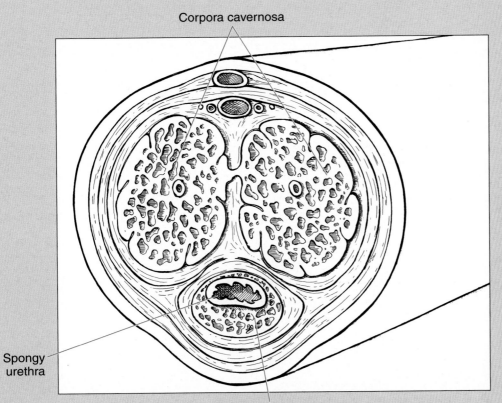

Corpora cavernosa

Figure 14-7 Cross section of the male penis.

Spongy
urethra

Corpus spongiosum

Some histological preparations of the penis are hemi-cross sections; therefore only part of the corpus spongiosum and spongy urethra and one of the two corpora cavernosa will be present. This photomicrograph (Figure 14-8) shows a hemisection of a human penis. Other slides used for penis specimens may have been obtained from animals possessing an os penis, as evidenced by the presence of bone (see section on Compact Bone—Cross Section—Ground Bone in Chapter 5) within the section. Keep these possibilities in mind as you examine your histological preparation.

Figure 14-8 is a photomicrograph of a segment of the wall from the *corpora cavernosa* within the human penis. The *corpora cavernosa* are surrounded by a dense capsule, termed the *tunica albuginea*. The tunica albuginea is composed of an inner circular and outer longitudinal layer of collagenous and elastic fibers. The interior of the body consists of a network of large spaces, or *lacunae*, lined by *endothelium* (termed *cavernous veins*) and separated by *fibrous trabeculae* rich in smooth muscle.

The *corpus spongiosum* is similar in structure to the corpora cavernosa. The corpus spongiosum, however, contains a higher density of elastic fibers and houses the *spongy urethra* (see section on Penis/Spongy Urethra in Chapter 12).

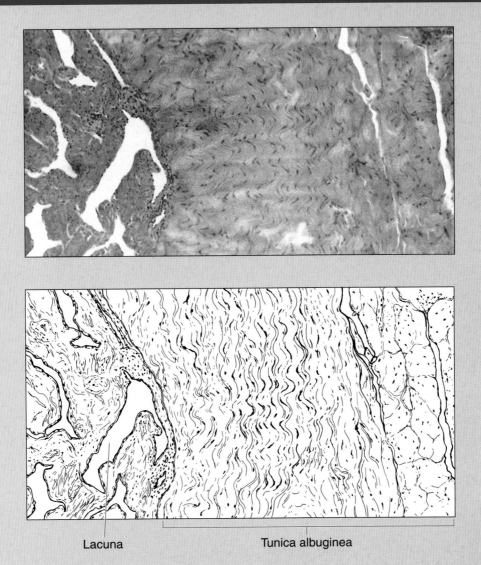

Lacuna   Tunica albuginea

Figure 14-8 (25×): Cross section of the human penis.

Prostate

The prostate may be separated into two regions: a central portion (including the urethra) that contains short glands and a more peripheral region containing slightly longer glands. The structures mentioned below may or may not be present in your preparation, depending on the plane of section.

A vascular, fibroelastic capsule with numerous smooth muscle fibers surrounds the prostate (Figures 14-9 and 14-10). (The capsule may not be present on your preparation.) From this capsule, broad *septa* radiate inward and become continuous with the abundant connective tissue of the interior of the prostate.

The stroma is fibromuscular, being a mix of smooth muscle and collagen fibers—a histological feature of the prostate.

The *glands of the prostate* (Figures 14-9 and 14-10) are lined with an epithelium that varies from low, simple columnar to pseudostratified columnar. The cells of the central region tend to be more irregular in height and more crowded when compared with the peripheral regions.

The ducts of the glands (which are not visible in these photomicrographs) possess a simple, columnar epithelium that will become transitional (see section on Transitional Epithelia in Chapter 2) near the junction of the *urethra*.

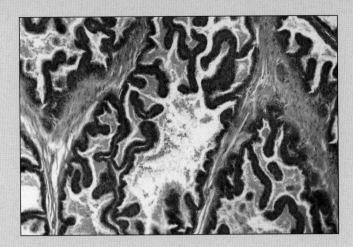

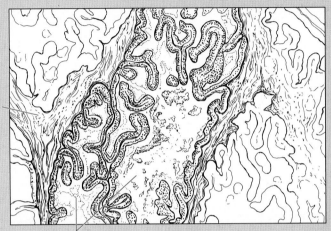

Figure 14-9 (25×): Prostate.

Septa

Glands of the prostate

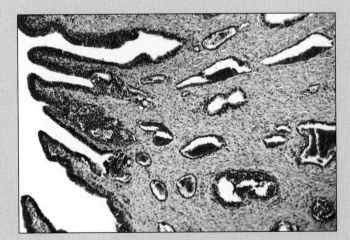

Figure 14-10 (25×): Prostate.

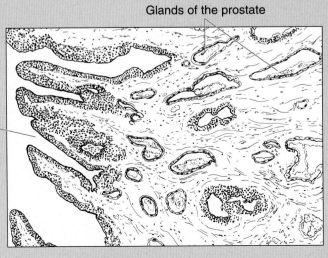

Glands of the prostate

Lumen
of urethra
(prostatic)

Ductus Deferens

The ductus deferens (vas deferens) possesses a thin *mucosa*, thick *muscularis*, and an outer *adventitia* (Figure 14-11).

The *epithelium* of the mucosa is a pseudostratified, columnar epithelium closely resembling that of the epididymis (see section on Efferent Ductules and the Epididymis in this chapter). However, unlike the epididymis, the mucosa of the ductus deferens is often thrown into longitudinal folds because of the contraction of underlying smooth muscle during fixation.

The *muscularis* of the ductus deferens consists of three layers of smooth muscle that are difficult to discern. These smooth muscle layers are arranged longitudinally (inner and outer layers) and circularly (middle layer).

Seminal Glands

The *mucosa* of the seminal glands (seminal vesicles) possesses numerous folds, which serve to increase the secretory surface area (Figure 14-12). The epithelium is a *pseudostratified, columnar epithelium* that may vary somewhat from location to location within the gland. The taller, nonciliated, columnar cells are secretory in nature, whereas the basal cells appear to be identical to those seen within other excretory ducts of the male reproductive system.

The *lamina propria* of the seminal gland forms the core of the primary and secondary mucosal folds, which extend into the *lumen* of the seminal glands.

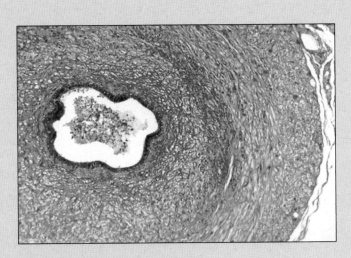

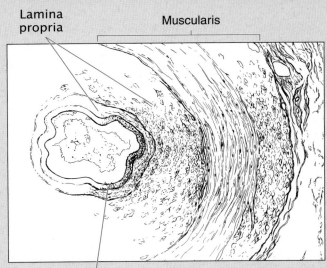

Lamina propria

Muscularis

Epithelium

Figure 14-11 (25×): Ductus deferens.

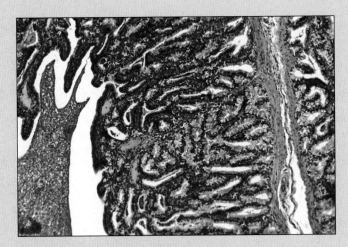

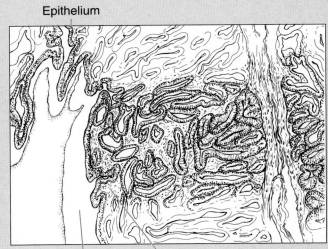

Epithelium

Lumen   Lamina propria

Figure 14-12 (25×): Seminal gland.

FEMALE REPRODUCTIVE SYSTEM

Components of the Female Reproductive System and Their Functions

The female reproductive system is composed of the following organs:

- External genitalia
- Vagina
- Uterus
- Uterine (Fallopian) tubes
- Ovaries
- Mammary glands

These organs serve a variety of functions, including the following. They:

- Produce the ova and prepare it for ovulation by the ovaries. In addition, the ovaries produce reproductive steroid hormones.

- Provide a passageway for sperm and ova between the uterus and ovaries by the uterine (Fallopian) tubes

- Provide an environment for blastocyst implantation and fetus development by the uterus. The uterus is also involved in placental development, expulsion of the fetus at birth, and the cyclical changes seen in the endometrium in response to varying blood levels of the hormones estrogen and progesterone.

- Produce and secrete milk

Ovary

The ovary is covered by a *simple squamous mesovarium*, termed the *surface epithelium* (Figure 15-1), which changes at the hilus (not visible in this photomicrograph) to a low, cuboidal epithelium (see section on the Classification of Epithelial Tissues in Chapter 2). Deep to the surface epithelium is the tunica albuginea, which is a dense, fibrous, connective tissue layer composed of collagenous and reticular fibers.

In cross section the ovary is composed of two zones: an inner *medulla* and an outer, broader *cortex* (Figure 15-1). The medulla is composed of a loose framework of connective tissue rich in elastin, blood vessels, lymphatics, and nerves. The cortex is composed of compact, richly cellular connective tissue in which *ovarian follicles* are scattered. There is no sharp demarcation line between the cortex and medulla.

The *cortex* of an ovary from a mature, premenopausal female will contain numerous follicles in varying stages of development and degeneration. The size and complexity of the follicle depends on the stage of development, yet each is composed of an oocyte surrounded by epithelial cells. Larger follicles also contain one or two connective tissue coats. The follicles of the ovary are divided into the following stages of development: primordial, primary, secondary (also termed *antral* or *growing*), and mature (*Graafian, ovulatory,* or *tertiary*).

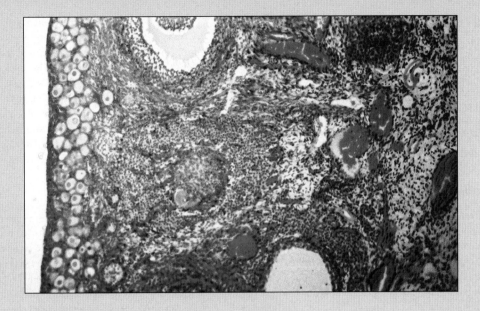

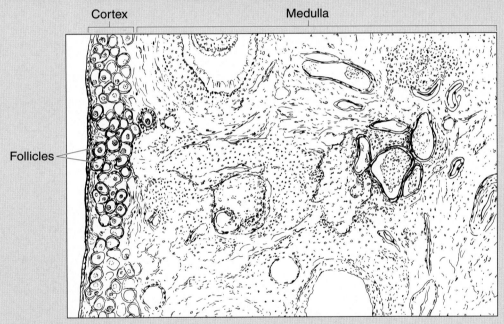

Figure 15-1 (25×): Ovary.

Primordial Follicles

Primordial follicles (Figure 15-2) are the most abundant and smallest of the follicles. Located at the periphery of the ovarian cortex, they consist of a *primary oocyte* surrounded by a few flattened *follicular cells.*

Primordial follicles are in a stage of arrested meiotic prophase and are unresponsive to hormones. Primordial follicles have been in this arrested stage of development since the fifth or sixth month of fetal development.

Primary Follicles

Primary follicles have started to grow, and changes are seen in the oocyte, follicular cells, and the adjacent connective tissue stroma. In an *early primary follicle* (Figure 15-2) the oocyte has started to enlarge, and the simple, squamous follicular cells enlarge to form a complete layer of cuboidal follicular cells around the oocyte. A basal lamina separates them from the rest of the ovary.

As the follicle continues to enlarge, it enters the *late primary phase* (Figure 15-3). In this phase, the oocyte continues to grow and secretes the *zona pellucida,* a glycoprotein coat that completely surrounds the oocyte. The follicular cells divide repeatedly, become multilayered, and are now called *granulosa cells.*

The *stromal cells* in the connective tissue surrounding the follicle have become organized into a distinct layer, the *theca interna.* The thecal cells are epithelioid in appearance and rounded in shape. They accumulate cytoplasmic lipid droplets that dissolve during the fixation process and are therefore quite pale staining.

Secondary Follicle

As the follicle continues to mature, it moves deeper into the cortical stroma of the ovary. In the *secondary follicle* (also termed an *antral follicle* or *maturing follicle*) (Figure 15-4), the *antrum,* a fluid-filled cavity, develops within the granulosa layer. The fluid within the antrum is called the *follicular fluid* (liquor folliculi). The antrum continues to enlarge in the secondary follicle.

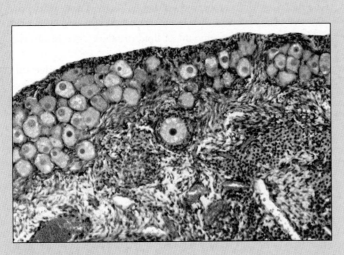

Primordial
follicles

Granulosa cells ⎤
Zona pellucida ⎦ Early primary follicle

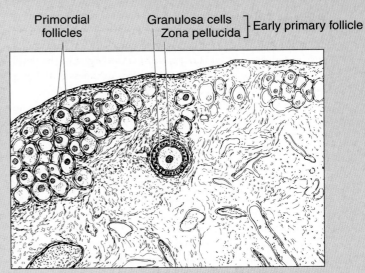

Figure 15-2 (50×): Primordial and early primary follicles within the ovary.

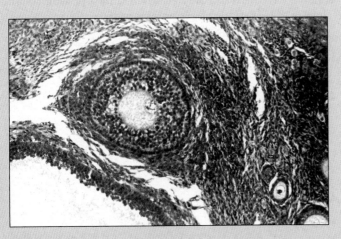

Granulosa cells　Zona pellucida　Theca interna

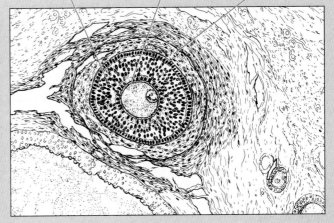

Figure 15-3 (50×): Late primary follicle within the ovary.

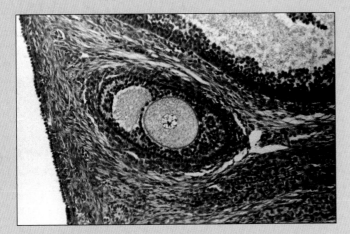

Antrum　Corona radiata

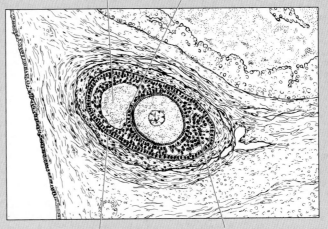

Granulosa cells　Follicular stalk

Figure 15-4 (50×): Secondary follicle within the ovary.

Mature Follicle

A *mature follicle* (also termed *preovulatory follicle, Graafian follicle* or *tertiary follicle*) (**Figure 15-5**) is the largest of the developing follicular stages, spanning the entire thickness of the ovarian cortex and causing a bulge on the surface of the ovary.

The mature follicle contains a large oocyte with a sizable nucleus and a prominent nucleolus (not visible in the current photomicrograph). The *zona pellucida* is now very thick, and the granulosa cells comprise a stratified epithelium with a basal layer that rests on a prominent basal lamina. The majority of the granulosa cells are small, with irregular cellular outlines, uniform nuclei, and numerous lipid droplets within the cytoplasm, giving the cells a light staining quality.

The antrum has enlarged and comes to occupy the majority of the follicle. As the antrum enlarged, the granulosa cells remained uniform in thickness, except for the region closest to the oocyte. These cells, which form the *cumulus oophorus*, project into the antrum and form the *follicular stalk*. The cells of the cumulus oophorus that completely surround the oocyte and that will remain with it at ovulation are termed the *corona radiata*.

As the mature follicle continues to prepare for ovulation, the corona radiata becomes only one cell thick, and the spaces between the granulosa cells enlarge. In addition, the oocyte and the cumulus oophorus cells gradually loosen from the rest of the granulosa cells. When ovulation occurs, the corona radiata and the loosely attached cells of the cumulus oophorus will remain with the oocyte.

In the mature follicle, the thecal layers have become even more prominent. The *theca interna* has thickened and now consists of a network of capillaries (see section on Capillaries in Chapter 8) with interspersed epithelioid cells. These cells possess the ultrastructure of steroid-secreting cells, and the cytoplasm contains a large amount of lipid droplets. As a result, the cells stain quite poorly.

The connective tissue surrounding the *theca interna* has differentiated and is now termed the *theca externa*. The theca externa is less vascular than the theca interna and possesses a larger number of collagenous fibers (see the discussion of collagenous fibers in the section on Loose, Irregular [Areolar] Connective Tissue in Chapter 3) and smooth muscle cells (see section on Smooth Muscle in Chapter 6).

Follicular Atresia

Numerous follicles in your specimen have undergone or are in the process of undergoing *follicular atresia* (**Figure 15-6**). This degenerative process can occur at any stage of follicular development.

Atresia of a primordial follicle is distinguished by the degeneration of the oocyte, indicated by a folding or general disintegration of its nucleus. On completion, atresia of a primordial follicle will leave little, if any, histological trace.

Atresia of a follicle in the primary stage or beyond is marked by hypertrophy of the thecal cells and autolysis of the granulosa cells, in addition to the degenerative changes observed within the oocyte discussed previously. The completion of follicular atresia is marked by a scar that represents the remnants of the zona pellucida.

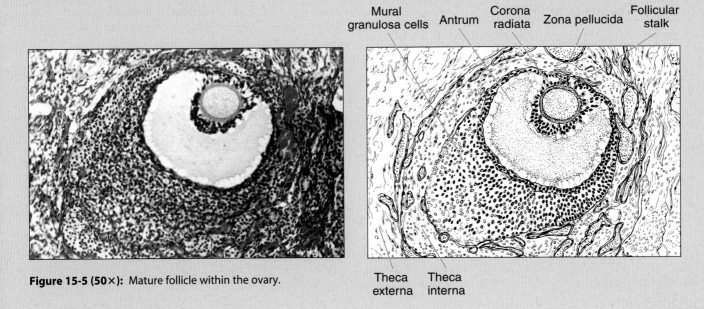

Figure 15-5 (50×): Mature follicle within the ovary.

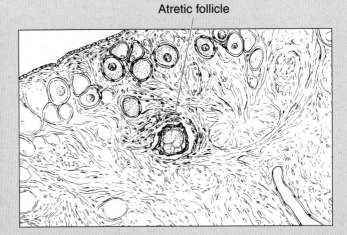

Figure 15-6 (50×): Follicular atresia.

Ovary/Corpus Luteum

Following ovulation and the subsequent release of the follicular fluid, the follicle collapses and becomes deeply infolded, thereby forming the *corpus luteum* (Figure 15-7). Cells of the theca interna and granulosa change morphologically, increasing in size and lipid content, and develop the ultrastructure of lipid-secreting cells.

Two cell types are identified within the corpus luteum. The greatest bulk of the corpus luteum is composed of *granulosa lutein cells*, which are differentiated from the granulosa cells. These are large, irregularly shaped cells with a centrally located nucleus and lightly staining cytoplasm.

The cells of the theca interna differentiate into *theca lutein cells* (also termed *paralutein cells*) (Figure 15-8). These will be seen along the folds and periphery of the corpus luteum. They are smaller and stain more darkly than the granulosa lutein cells.

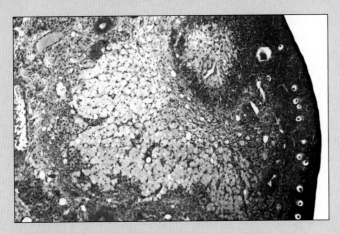

Figure 15-7 (50×): Corpus luteum within the ovary.

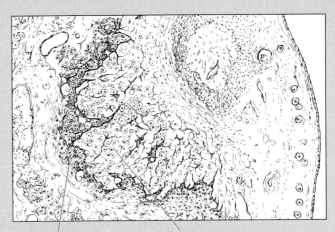

Theca lutein cells   Granulosa lutein cells

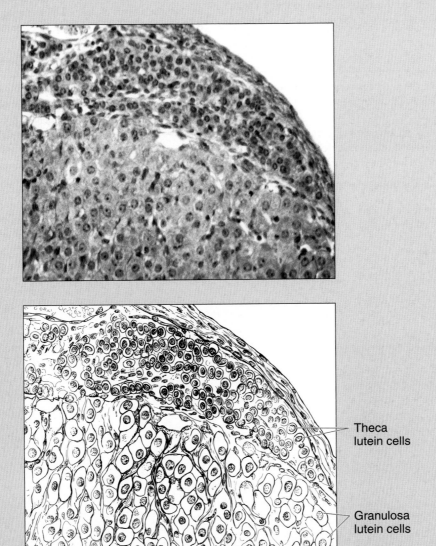

Theca
lutein cells

Granulosa
lutein cells

Figure 15-8 (100×): Corpus luteum within the ovary.

Uterine Tubes

The uterine tubes (*oviducts* or *Fallopian tubes*) are composed of three regions: infundibulum, ampulla, and isthmus. The walls of the uterine tubes are composed of three layers: an inner *mucosa*, middle *muscularis*, and outer *serosa*.

As you can see in **Figures** 15-9 and 15-10, the *mucosa* is folded to a variable extent. These folds will decrease in height as you progress toward the uterus. The epithelium of the mucosa is simple columnar (see section on Simple Columnar Epithelium in Chapter 2), with some of the cells possessing cilia. The lamina propria in the isthmus of the uterine tube is quite cellular because it is composed of loose, irregular (areolar) connective tissue.

The *muscularis* is composed of an inner circular and an outer longitudinal layer of smooth muscle. The thickness of the muscularis layer will vary, depending on the source of your specimen, with the muscularis in the isthmic region being thicker than that of the ampulla even though the longitudinal layer is less prominent.

The serosa (not visible on this photomicrograph) is a typical peritoneal structure.

Uterus

The wall of the body of the uterus is composed of three layers, the outermost of which is the peritoneum, not visible on this photomicrograph.

The second layer is the *myometrium* (**Figure 15-11**), which is composed of three layers of smooth muscle. The inner layer is longitudinally arranged and is termed the *submucosal layer (sub-vascular stratum)*. The *vascular layer* comprises the second, circularly arranged layer, which forms the bulk of the myometrium. The outermost layer of the myometrium is called the *supravascular layer* and is a relatively thin layer of smooth muscle fibers that are circularly and longitudinally arranged. (Note: The inner longitudinal layer of the supravascular layer is absent from the cervix of the uterus.)

Between the smooth muscle layers you will see loosely arranged collagenous and elastic fibers and relatively few connective tissue cells (see section on the cells of Loose, Irregular [Areolar] Connective Tissue in Chapter 3). The connective tissue may be especially evident in the outermost portion of the muscularis.

The innermost layer of the uterus is a mucous membrane termed the *endometrium*. The luminal surface of the endometrium is lined by a simple columnar epithelium, with some of the cells possessing cilia. The epithelium has numerous branched and coiled tubular *glands* within it. The length of the glands indicates the depth of the endometrium. The remainder of the endometrium is composed of an extremely cellular connective tissue stroma.

The endometrium undergoes considerable histological changes during the menstrual cycle, and the most superficial portion is lost if implantation does not occur. The part of the endometrium that is lost during menstruation is termed the *functional layer* (also termed the *decidua functionalis*); the part that is retained is termed the *basal layer (decidua basalis)*. The basal layer is the deepest portion of the endometrium and may stain more basophilic than the functional layer on your preparation.

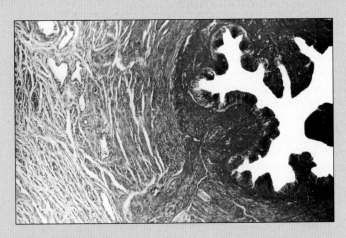

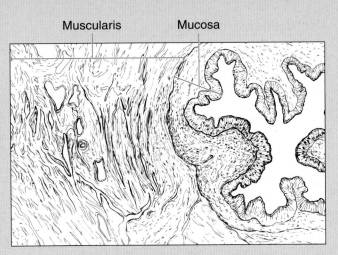

Muscularis   Mucosa

Figure 15-9 (25×): Uterine tube.

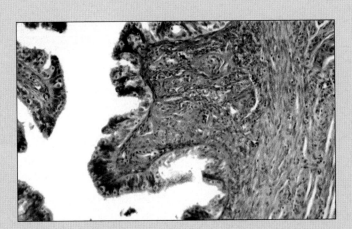

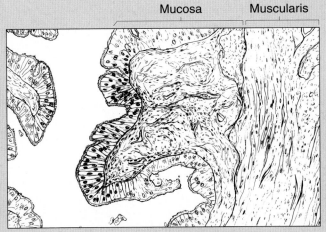

Mucosa   Muscularis

Figure 15-10 (50×): Uterine tube.

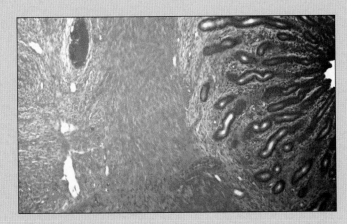

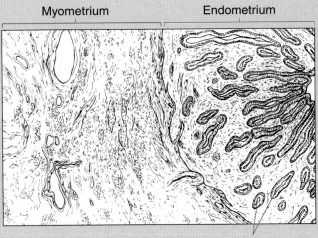

Myometrium   Endometrium

Glands

Figure 15-11 (25×): Uterus.

Uterus/Menstrual Cycle

Uterus/Proliferative Phase

The proliferative phase (also termed *follicular* or *early postmenstrual phase*) is a period of rapid regeneration of the endometrium (Figure 15-12). The epithelial cells of the *glands* of the basal layer are rapidly undergoing mitosis, and the resulting daughter cells are spreading over the remaining stromal cells to reestablish the *luminal epithelium*. As a result, the epithelial layer is a particularly thin, simple columnar epithelium. Mitotic figures may be present within both the luminal epithelium and stroma of the uterus. *The uterine glands of the proliferative stage tend to be rather narrow, straight, and short—a major histological feature of this stage.*

Uterus/Ovulatory Phase

In the ovulatory phase of the cycle (second week postmenstrual, early luteal, or presecretory) (Figure 15-13) *the epithelium becomes pseudostratified columnar* (see section on Pseudostratified Epithelia in Chapter 2) *and the glands become longer and larger in diameter. Because of their increased length and corkscrew shape, cross and tangential sections of the glands will become more frequent within the endometrium. Both of these are important histological features of this phase of the menstrual cycle.*

Late in this phase of the cycle, edema starts to develop within the connective tissue stroma; therefore the connective tissue within the functional layer stains less homogeneously. However, the staining characteristics of the basal layer tend to remain relatively constant throughout this phase. The endometrium increases in size overall, reaching 75% or more of its maximal size during this phase of the cycle.

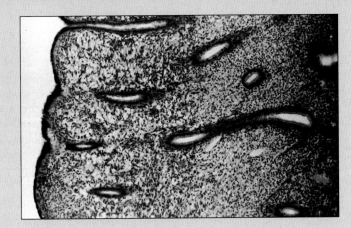

Figure 15-12 (25×): Menstrual cycle of the uterus: Proliferative phase.

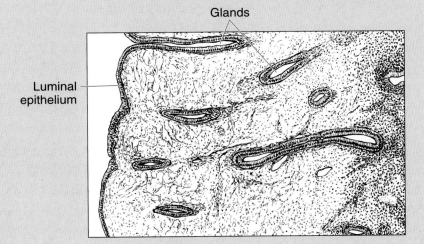

Glands

Luminal epithelium

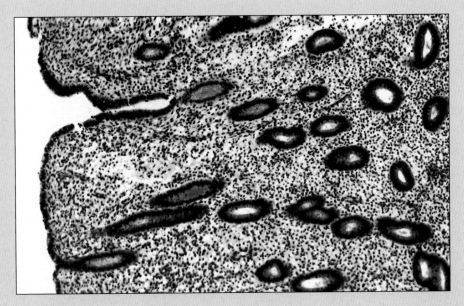

Figure 15-13 (25×): Menstrual cycle of the uterus: Ovulatory phase.

Uterus/Secretory (Late Luteal) Phase

The endometrium continues to increase in thickness during the secretory phase (late luteal phase) (Figure 15-14). *The glands have now reached their maximal length and have developed the characteristically saw-toothed appearance. The glycogen content within the cells increases such that late in the secretory phase the nuclei become apically located. Both of these histological features are important in making a correct identification of this phase of the menstrual cycle.*

Uterus/Menstrual Phase

In this phase of the cycle, the decidualization (sloughing off) of the stromal cells occurs in the superficial parts of the endometrium (Figure 15-15).

Early in this phase, the basal layer is further subdivided into the superficial stratum compactum and the deeper stratum spongiosum. With the onset of menstruation, *red blood cells* and leukocytes are present within the stroma and lumen. The endometrium is considerably reduced in thickness because of the loss of the most superficial portions of the stratum functionale.

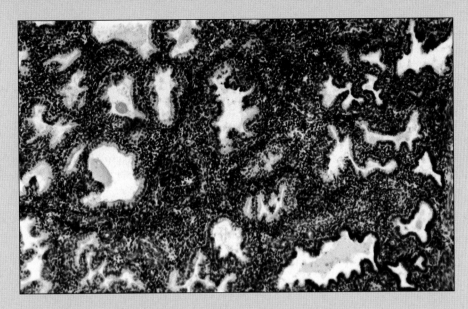

Figure 15-14 (25×): Menstrual cycle of the uterus: Secretory phase.

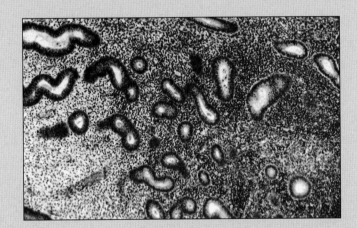

Figure 15-15 (25×): Menstrual cycle of the uterus: Menstrual phase.

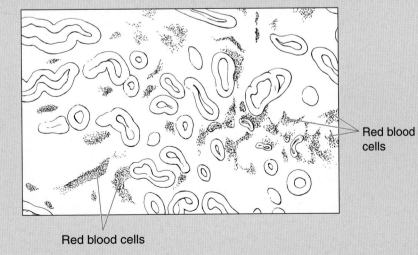

Red blood cells

Red blood cells

Vagina

The wall of the vagina consists of three layers, the innermost of which is the *mucosa* (**Figure 15-16**), which demonstrates transversely orientated folds *(rugae)*. The lumen of the vagina is lined by a *nonkeratinized, stratified, squamous epithelium (mucosal type)* (see section on Stratified Squamous Epithelium [Mucosal Type] in Chapter 2) resting on a prominent basal lamina and an underlying lamina propria. The appearance of lymphocytes and leukocytes is quite common within the lamina propria.

The muscularis of the vagina is made up of bundles of longitudinally and circumferentially arranged smooth muscle. *This orientation of the muscularis may serve as a major histological feature of the vagina.* Bundles of connective tissue rich in elastic fibers separate the muscle layers.

The outermost layer of the vagina is the adventitia, which is not visible on this photomicrograph. The adventitia is composed of loose, irregular (areolar) connective tissue rich in elastic fibers.

Lactating Mammary Gland

A superficial layer of subcutaneous fat (not visible in this photomicrograph) covers the entire organ, except for the nipple and surrounding the areola.

Each mammary gland is composed of 15 to 20 lobules (**Figure 15-17**). Each lobule is a compound gland with a separate *lobular duct*, which is lined by simple cuboidal epithelium. The lobular duct opens at the apex of the nipple.

During lactation, the tubules characteristic of an inactive gland form buds that enlarge into secretory *alveoli*, all of which are connected to a duct. Many of these alveoli appear as oval or spherical profiles lined by secretory cells arranged into a simple cuboidal epithelium.

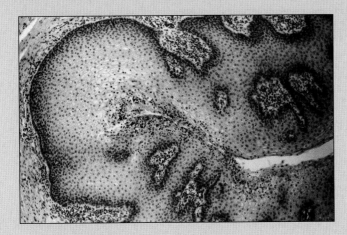

Figure 15-16 (25×): Vagina.

Lamina propria

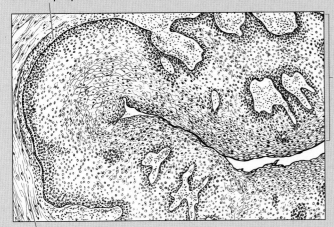

Epithelium

Muscularis

Alveoli   Ducts

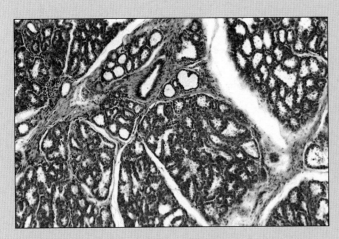

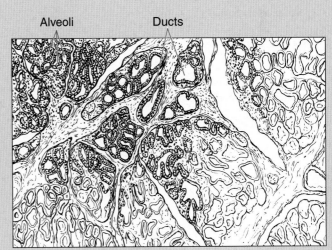

Figure 15-17 (25×): Lactating mammary gland.

Commonly Misidentified Tissues

Lactating Mammary Gland and Thyroid Gland

When identifying various sections of the female reproductive system, several common mistakes are made. It is not uncommon to confuse a lactating mammary gland and the thyroid gland, or to mistake the corpus luteum for the adrenal cortex. Therefore you should keep the following histological features in mind:

Lactating Mammary Gland (Review **Figure 15-17** in section on the Lactating Mammary Gland)

1. There are ducts connected to each alveolus.

2. Gland is clearly lobulated.

3. Secretion within alveoli appears granulated.

4. Alveoli are irregular in shape.

Thyroid Gland (Review **Figures 13-5** and **13-6** in section on the Thyroid Gland in Chapter 13)

1. There is an absence of ducts.

2. Lobulation is lacking.

3. Colloid within follicles stains more homogeneously.

Corpus Luteum and Adrenal Gland

Corpus Luteum (Review **Figures 15-7** and **15-8** in section on the Ovary and Corpus Luteum)

1. Developing follicles present within section when viewed under low or medium power

2. Arrangement of cells into homogeneous cords within the gland

3. Absence of capsule

Adrenal Gland (Review **Figures 13-9–13-12** in section on the Suprarenal [Adrenal] Gland in Chapter 13)

1. Cells are arranged into cortex and medulla when viewed under low or medium power.

2. Cells of cortex are arranged into three layers.

Ureter and Isthmic Region of the Uterine Tubes

Another common misidentification, even among experienced histologists, involves the ureter and isthmic region of the uterine (Fallopian) tubes. Both of these structures have a convoluted lumen surrounded by a considerable amount of smooth muscle. In trying to differentiate between these two structures, you should keep in mind the following differences:

Ureter (Review **Figure 12-8** in section on the Ureter in Chapter 12)

1. Transitional epithelium

2. Muscularis arranged with an inner longitudinal layer and an outer circular layer

3. Star-shaped lumen

Isthmic Region of Uterine Tubes (Review **Figures 15-9** and **15-10** in section on the Uterine Tubes)

1. Simple cuboidal epithelium (some possessing cilia)

2. Highly folded mucosa

3. Muscularis arranged with an inner circular layer and an outer longitudinal layer

Chapter 16

GASTROINTESTINAL SYSTEM

Chapter Objectives

This chapter will enable you to identify and discuss the histological:

1. Characteristics of the lips

2. Structure of the tongue and the circumvallate papillae and associated taste buds

3. Characteristics of the tubuloacinar glands of the salivary glands and the general characteristics of each form of salivary gland

4. Characteristics of the esophagus and how these characteristics change with the level of sectioning

5. Changes that occur in the hollow organs of the gastrointestinal tract as you progress from the esophagus to the large intestine and appendix

6. Forms of mucosal glands of the stomach

7. Regional specializations of the small intestine

8. Characteristics of the colon

9. Characteristics of the appendix and gallbladder

10. Characteristics of the pancreas and liver

General Organization of the Hollow Organs of the Digestive System

The gastrointestinal (GI) system is composed of the hollow gastrointestinal tract and associated accessory structures (teeth, salivary glands, tongue, liver, gallbladder, and pancreas). The hollow organs, starting at the esophagus, share a common, general organization. With few exceptions, these organs are arranged into four layers. From superficial to deep, these layers and their general characteristics are as follows:

- Mucosa

  - Composed of an epithelium sitting on a connective tissue lamina propria

  - May possess a layer of smooth muscle deep to the lamina propria, which is termed the *lamina muscularis* of the mucosa in the esophagus and *muscularis mucosae* throughout the remainder of the hollow organs of the digestive tract

- Submucosa

  - Composed of irregular connective tissue

  - Found deep to the lamina propria and lamina muscularis

  - Starts at the level of the esophagus and is found in all hollow organs of the GI system except the gallbladder

- Muscularis Externa

  - Typically composed of two layers of smooth muscle (inner circular and outer longitudinal)

  - May also include visceral striated muscle, as in the esophagus, or may include a third layer of smooth muscle, as in the stomach

- Serosa (adventitia)

  - Composed of mesothelium and connective tissue or connective tissue only (as in the esophagus)

Lips

Figure 16-1 is a hematoxylin and eosin (H & E) preparation of human lips. On scanning power, note the region of transition in the thickness of the epithelium. This is the *transitional area* (also termed the *vermilion part*) from the cutaneous (facial or exterior) part of the lip to the mucosal (oral cavity or interior) part. The *cutaneous part* consists of a keratinized, stratified squamous epithelium (see section on Stratified Squamous Keratinized Epithelium in Chapter 2) resting on a prominent layer of connective tissue. Within the connective tissue you may find sweat glands, sebaceous glands, and the bases of hair follicles.

The transition from the cutaneous part to the *mucosal part* is marked by the following characteristics:

- A gradual thickening of the epithelium

- A gradual disappearance of keratinized cells and a transition to a stratified squamous epithelium (mucosal type)

- A gradual increase in the height of the connective tissue papillae

- The disappearance of hair follicles, sebaceous and sweat glands

- The appearance of labial (mixed or seromucous) glands in the connective tissue deep to the mucosal surface

Tongue and Vallate Papillae

A thick layer of *stratified squamous epithelium* covers the tongue **(Figure 16-2)**. The upper surface is studded with projections known as *lingual papillae*. Deep to the epithelium is the *lamina propria* (also termed the *tunica propria*), which is composed of areolar connective tissue (see section on Loose, Irregularly Arranged [Areolar] Connective Tissue in Chapter 3). This connective tissue forms the core of the papillae.

The *musculature of the tongue* is composed of skeletal muscle (see section on Skeletal Muscle in Chapter 6) arranged into three interlacing layers: vertical, transverse, and longitudinal. Among these bundles, you will note considerable amounts of fibroelastic connective tissue with varying numbers of blood vessels (see section on Blood Vessels in Chapter 8), peripheral nerves (see section on Peripheral nerves in Chapter 7), and adipose cells (see section on White Adipose Tissue in Chapter 3). Seromucous glands (see discussion of compound tubuloacinar glands in the section on the Parotid Salivary Gland in Chapter 2) may also be present on your specimen (not visible in this photomicrograph).

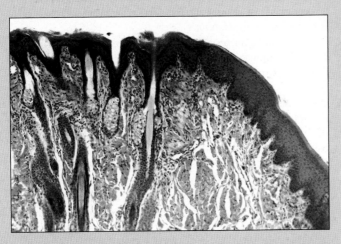

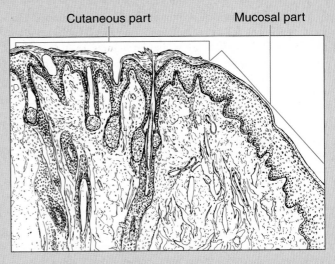

Cutaneous part   Mucosal part

Figure 16-1 (25×): Lip.

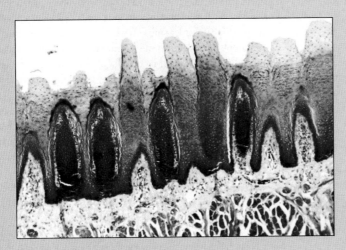

Figure 16-2 (25×): Tongue.

Lingual papillae

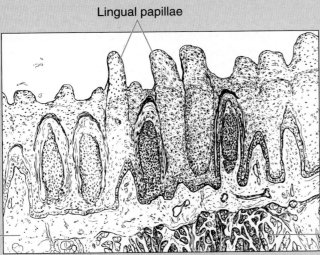

Lamina propria

Skeletal muscle

Four forms of papillae are found on the human tongue: filiform, fungiform, foliate, and vallate (also termed *circumvallate*) papillae. *Vallate papillae* are visible on Figures 16-3 and 16-4. They are rather large, dome-shaped papillae and are surrounded by a moat-like furrow. The papillae and furrow are covered by a noncornified, stratified squamous epithelium.

Taste buds are found on the lateral surface of the papillae and the outer wall of the furrow. Taste buds are little, barrel-shaped groups of cells embedded in the papillae. Each taste bud is connected to the surface by a small opening, the *gustatory pore*, which may not be visible on your specimen. Two of the following three cell types that make up a taste bud are visible in Figure 16-4:

- *Supporting* (sustentacular) *cells* are elongated cells with a slender, darker staining nucleus.

- *Gustatory* (neuroepithelial, taste or sensory) *cells* exhibit a lighter, more oval nucleus and cytoplasm that may or may not stain lighter.

- Basal epithelial cells are located at the periphery of the taste bud and possess an elongated, darker-staining nucleus and are not visible in this photomicrograph.

Salivary Glands

A number of different types of salivary glands secrete into the oral cavity. For convenience, these are subdivided into two groups: minor salivary glands and major salivary glands. The minor salivary glands secrete continuously and contribute to the saliva of the oral cavity. They open onto the oral mucosa either directly or via short ducts.

The major salivary glands include the parotid, submandibular, and sublingual salivary glands. They release their secretions in response to mechanical, olfactory, or neural stimuli. These glands are located some distance from the oral epithelium and are connected to it by a series of branching ducts. The secretory cells of the major salivary glands are arranged into glandular acini.

Except for the parotid, the major salivary glands are mixed glands. The secretory portions are ovoid or elongated acini at the ends of a duct. In these mixed glands, some acini are made up exclusively of serous cells and others are composed entirely of mucous cells. Other acini consist of mucous cells capped by a crescent layer of serous cells. This arrangement of secretory cells is termed a *serous demilune*.

In mucous acini, a single layer of plump, pyramidal cells rests on a basal lamina. The cytoplasm of these cells is filled with pale droplets of mucigen. During histological preparation the droplets of mucigen are partially or totally extracted, leaving round, clear areas outlined by a thin network of cytoplasm. The nucleus is displaced far to the base of the cell and may be deformed by the accumulated secretory product that occupies the greater part of the volume of the cell.

In serous acini, the cells have a columnar or truncated pyramidal form and surround a smaller lumen than that seen in mucous acini. The apical portion of the cell is crowded with secretory granules, thereby giving the cells a granular appearance. Cells of serous acini stain richly basophilic and are protein-secreting cells.

Acini containing both serous and mucous cells were traditionally called *seromucous acini*. This term is no longer used because it was discovered that some cells secrete both protein and carbohydrate products. To eliminate any possible confusion, acini containing both serous and mucous cells are now called *mixed acini*. In this type of acinus, both types of cells are segregated. The mucous cells occupy the proximal end of the acinus and the serous cells are displaced to the distal end, where they appear as a crescent cap of dark-staining cells, the serous demilune. The cells of the serous demilune appear to be separated from the lumen of the acinus by the underlying mucous cells. However, the secretions from the serous demilune are conducted to the lumen of the acinus through narrow channels between the mucous cells. These narrow channels are visible with the electron microscope but not with the light microscope.

Salivary ducts have varying diameters. Smaller-diameter intercalated ducts have a small lumen and are lined by a simple cuboidal epithelium. These ducts empty into larger-diameter striated ducts, which are lined by simple columnar epithelial cells with basal infoldings, thereby pushing the nucleus into the upper half of the cell. Interlobular ducts are lined by epithelium that may be simple columnar in the smaller-diameter interlobular ducts or pseudostratified columnar or stratified columnar in the larger-diameter interlobular ducts.

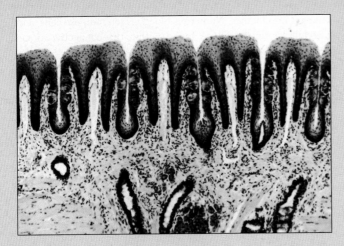

Figure 16-3 (25×): Vallate papillae of the tongue.

Vallate papilla

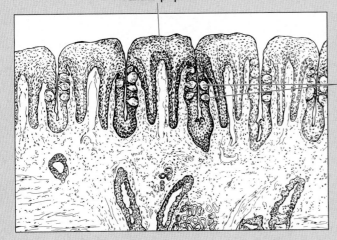

Taste buds

Basal cell   Gustatory cell   Sustentacular cell

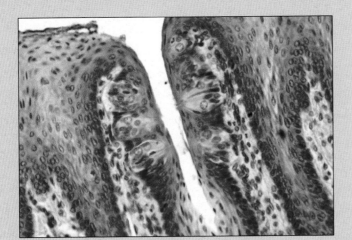

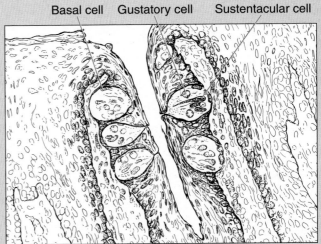

Figure 16-4 (25×): Vallate papillae of the tongue.

Parotid Salivary Gland

The parotid salivary gland is classified as a *serous gland* (Figure 16-5). It is surrounded by a connective tissue capsule that sends numerous *septa* into the interior of the gland, subdividing it into lobules. Numerous blood vessels, adipose cells, and interlobular ducts will be found within the connective tissue septa between the lobules.

Within each lobule (**Figure 16-6**) are numerous *serous acini*, isolated *adipose cells*, and *striated ducts*.

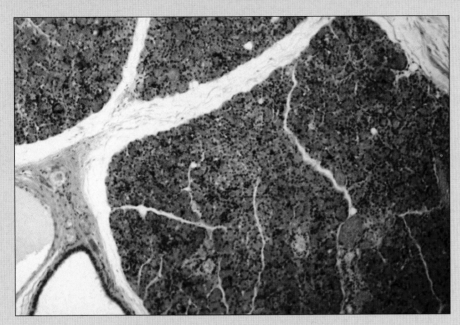

Figure 16-5 (25×): Parotid salivary gland.

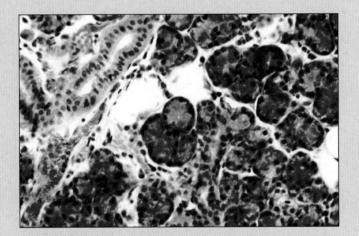

Figure 16-6 (100×): Parotid salivary gland.

Duct   Serous acinus

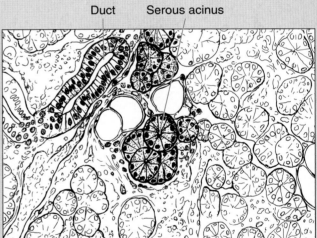

Submandibular Salivary Gland

The submandibular gland (Figure 16-7) is a compound, mixed tubuloacinar gland because it is composed of *mucous* and *serous* acini. *Serous acini dominate within this gland. Serous demilunes* are visible within this photomicrograph.

Sublingual Salivary Gland

Like the submandibular salivary gland, the sublingual salivary gland (Figure 16-8) is a compound, mixed tubuloacinar gland composed of *mucous* and *serous* acini. However, *most of the secretory acini within this salivary gland are mucous in nature.*

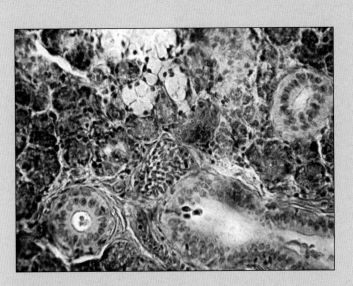

Serous acini   Mucous acinus   Mucous acinus with serous demilune

Figure 16-7 (50×): Submandibular salivary gland.

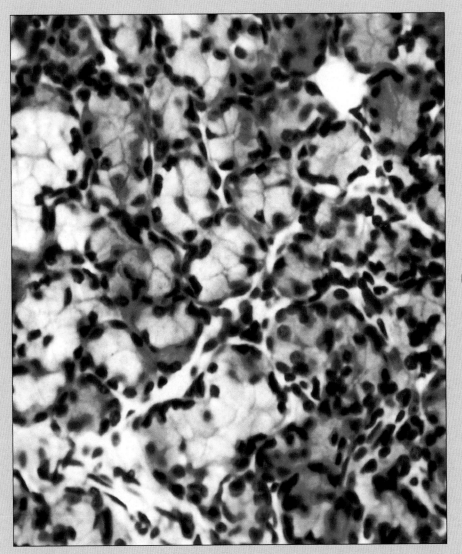

Figure 16-8 (100×): Sublingual salivary gland.

Esophagus

Note: The following descriptions and photomicrographs are of the human esophagus. The mucosa and muscularis externa will vary in specimens obtained from other animals.

The *mucosa* of the esophagus (Figure 16-9) is composed of a stratified squamous epithelium (mucosal type). The *lamina propria* is quite prominent and is interspersed with fibroblasts, fibrocytes, and macrophages (see sections on Loose, Irregularly Arranged [Areolar] Connective Tissue [mesenteric spread and lamina propria of duodenum] in Chapter 3).

The *lamina muscularis* (Figure 16-9) is composed mostly of longitudinally arranged smooth muscle fibers but may possess some circularly arranged fibers (see section on Smooth Muscle in Chapter 6). *Esophageal glands* are found within the lamina propria of the mucosa. *Superior esophageal glands* (which may be absent in some specimens) are found in the superior (uppermost) region of the esophagus (Figure 16-9), whereas *esophageal cardiac glands* are found in the inferior region (see Figure 16-11). Structurally, the esophageal cardiac glands are similar to those found within the cardiac region of the stomach.

The *submucosa* (Figures 16-9–16-11), which is composed of loose, irregularly arranged (areolar) connective tissue, may contain *submucosal glands*, blood vessels, lymphatics, and occasionally autonomic nervous system ganglia. Question: These ganglia belong to which branch of the autonomic nervous system and why?

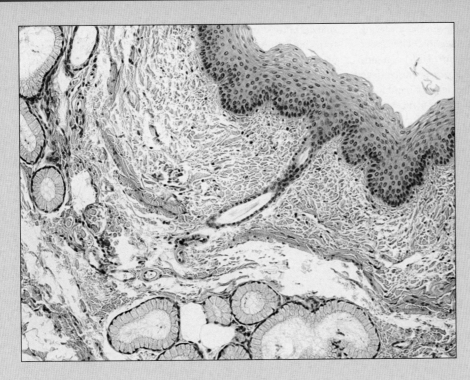

Figure 16-9 (25×): Esophagus (upper one third).

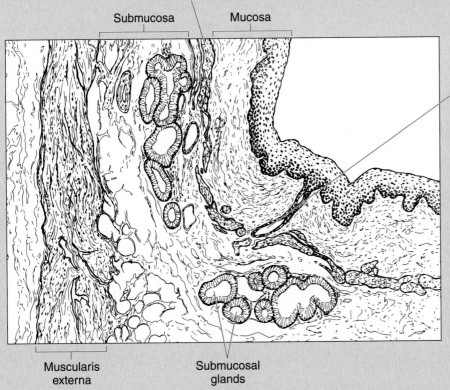

Muscularis mucosae

Submucosa   Mucosa

Esophageal gland

Muscularis externa

Submucosal glands

The *muscularis externa* of the human esophagus has a varying composition, depending on the level of the section. The upper one fourth to one third of the esophagus **(Figure 16-9)** contains a muscularis externa composed of *visceral striated muscle* (see classification of two types of Skeletal Muscle in Chapter 6), whereas the middle one-third **(Figure 16-10)** is a mixture of *smooth muscle* and *visceral striated muscle.* The muscularis externa in the lower one third **(Figure 16-11)** is composed entirely of *smooth muscle.*

The adventitia (not visible in this photomicrograph) is composed of loose, irregularly arranged (areolar) connective tissue.

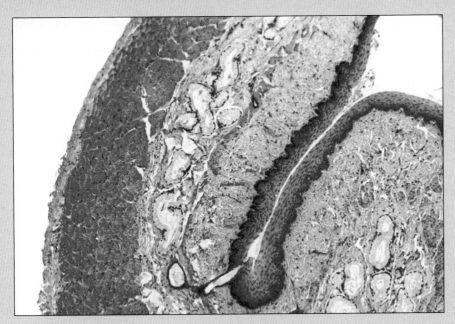

Figure 16-10 (25×): Esophagus (middle one third).

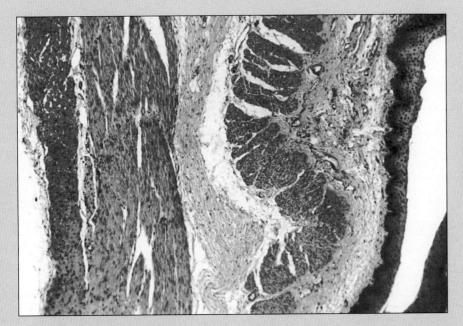

Figure 16-11 (25×): Esophagus (lower one third).

Stomach

Cardio-Esophageal Junction

Figure 16-12 shows the junction of the esophagus and stomach. This photomicrograph clearly demonstrates the abrupt histological changes that occur at the junction of the two organs. In the human esophagus, the mucosal epithelium is stratified squamous and rests on a lamina propria containing numerous papillae, whereas the mucosa of the stomach contains a surface of simple columnar epithelium and numerous tubular glands resting on a highly cellular lamina propria.

At the junction of these two organs, the lowest layer of cells from the esophageal mucosa continues on into the mucosa of the stomach. On examination of this junction during gross dissection of an unpreserved cadaver, you would see the whitish epithelium of the esophagus change into the bright pink of the stomach. This pink color is due to the superficial location of blood vessels within the lamina propria and the thinness of the epithelium.

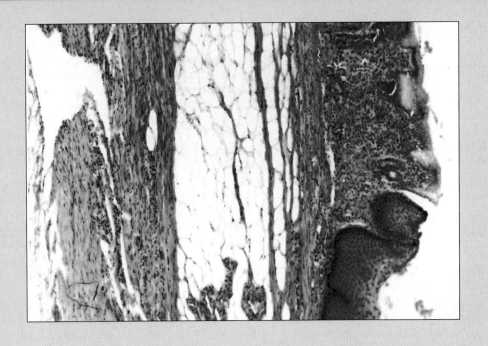

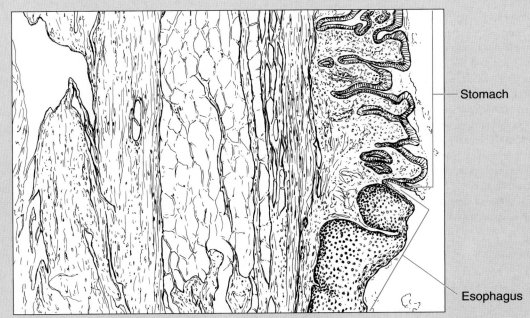

Figure 16-12 (25×): Cardioesophageal junction.

General Histological Description of the Stomach

As you read the general histology of the stomach, you should examine all of the figures in this section because some items listed in italics may be seen better in one region than another or may be seen only in a particular region of the stomach. Subsequent discussions compare the histological differences among the cardiac, fundic, and pyloric regions of the stomach.

As you examine the histology of the stomach, you should direct your attention to two main questions:

1. What histological characteristics will differentiate the stomach from other hollow organs of the gastrointestinal tract?

2. What histological characteristics will allow you to differentiate among the different regions of the stomach?

Start your examination of the stomach with **Figure 16-13.** On gross examination of the stomach you would see that the *mucosa* of the stomach possesses numerous *gastric folds* (also termed *gastric rugae*). In addition to the folds, the epithelium is subdivided into smaller grooves termed *gastric* (or *mamillated*) areas. These gastric areas are studded with minute depressions termed *gastric pits*.

The *epithelium* lining the inner surface of the stomach and gastric pits is composed of *simple, columnar, mucous surface cells* that differ structurally and functionally from those of the gastric glands. The apical end of the cells has a deep, cup-shaped zone filled with mucigen, which is not preserved in routine histological sections, thereby giving the cells a clear apical end. The single nucleus is oval or spheroidal in shape, depending on the shape of the cell and the amount of mucigen present. Short microvilli may be present on the apical surface of the cell but are not readily visible with the light microscope. As these cells extend deeper into the gastric pits, they become progressively shorter and possess less mucigen.

The *lamina propria* consists of a delicate interweaving of loose, irregularly arranged (areolar) connective tissue. This region of the mucosa contains the *gastric glands, a major histological feature of the stomach.* The glands are so numerous that the lamina propria and associated connective tissue fibers are reduced to thin strands. Scattered lymphoid nodules may be present within the lamina propria.

The *muscularis mucosae* are composed of a thin layer of circularly and longitudinally arranged smooth muscle.

The *submucosa* consists of dense, irregular connective tissue. Large blood vessels and nerve plexuses may be seen in some sections. (Note: The submucosa in **Figure 16-13** is altered significantly by a fixation and sectioning artifact.)

The muscularis externa is a major histological feature of the stomach. It is composed of three separate layers of smooth muscle: inner oblique, middle circular, and outer longitudinal layers. Connective tissue separates these layers, and autonomic nervous system ganglia may be found between the three layers of smooth muscle.

The serosa consists of a layer of loose, irregularly arranged (areolar) connective tissue covered by a simple squamous mesothelium and typically is not visible in histological sections.

Beginning histology students must understand the variation in terminology between the gross anatomy of the stomach and the histological anatomy of the stomach. Gross anatomists divide the stomach into four regions: (1) cardia, or that portion found at the junction between the esophagus and the stomach; (2) fundus, the portion of the stomach that is superior to a horizontal line drawn at the junction of the esophagus and the cardia of the stomach; (3) body, that region found inferior to this horizontal line; and (4) pylorus, the narrow segment found at the junction between the stomach and the duodenum. Histologists, however, divide the stomach into only three regions, based on the type of glands found within a particular region of the stomach: (1) cardiac region, which is that region of the stomach possessing cardiac glands; (2) fundic region, the portion of the stomach containing fundic glands; and (3) pyloric region, that region of the stomach possessing pyloric glands.

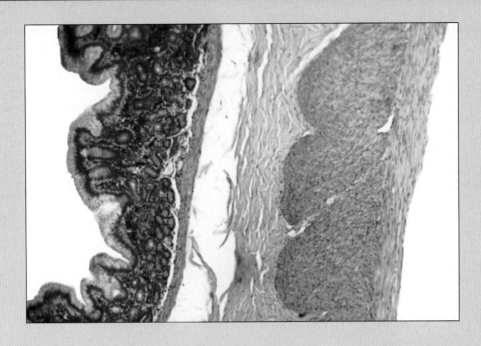

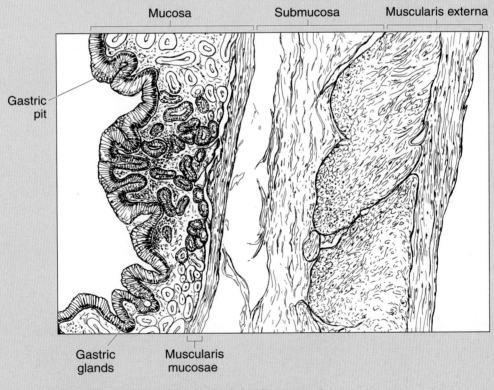

Figure 16-13 (25×): General histology of the stomach.

Cardiac Stomach

Figure 16-14 is of the cardiac region of the stomach. *The surface epithelium and the composition of the glands are major histological features of this region of the stomach.* The surface epithelium is a simple columnar epithelium (see section on the Simple Columnar Epithelium in Chapter 2) composed of *surface mucous cells. The glands of the cardiac stomach are typically shorter than those seen in the fundic or pyloric regions.* In addition, the glands of this region are composed mainly of *mucous neck cells.* The staining intensity of the mucous surface cells and mucous neck cells will vary, ranging from acidophilic to clear, depending on the amount of mucous that was present in the cell at the time of fixation.

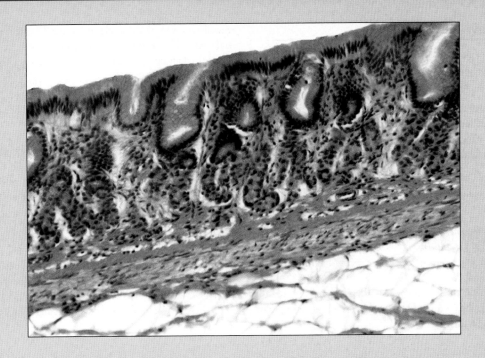

Surface mucous cells   Mucous neck cell

Figure 16-14 (50×): Cardiac stomach.

Fundic Stomach

The transition between the cardiac and fundic regions is gradual. Histologically, the fundic stomach differs from the cardiac and pyloric regions in at least two ways **(Figures 16-15 and 16-16):**

- The arrangement of the muscularis externa: In the fundus the muscle bundles do not run in discrete layers; rather, they course in various directions, making the differentiation of three distinct bundles quite difficult.

- The histological appearance and cellular makeup of the gastric glands, which are termed *fundic glands*, differs significantly from that of the cardiac and pyloric regions.

Of these two differences, the ability to recognize the histological characteristics of the fundic glands will yield the most consistent results when you are trying to differentiate among the three regions of the stomach.

The *fundic glands* **(Figure 16-15)** are straight or slightly branched and extend downward through the entire thickness of the lamina propria to the muscularis mucosae. Three-dimensional reconstruction of these glands shows that three to seven individual gastric glands empty into a single gastric pit. Three cell types typically can be distinguished in the glands **(Figure 16-16):**

- *Chief cells* are the most numerous types of cells in the fundic glands. They are large, pyramidal cells with a single, basally located nucleus. The cytoplasm stains lightly basophilic.

- *Parietal cells* are often larger than chief cells and often found in the upper one third of the gland. They are oval or polygonal in shape. The nucleus is centrally located within the cell; binucleated or multinucleated cells are not uncommon. The cytoplasm is granular in appearance and stains well with acidophilic stains.

- The third cell type is the *mucous neck cell*. These are found interspersed among the parietal cells. They are cuboidal or low columnar in shape and contain a basally situated nucleus and finely granular cytoplasm. Mucous neck cells stain more lightly than chief cells but not as lightly as the surface epithelium.

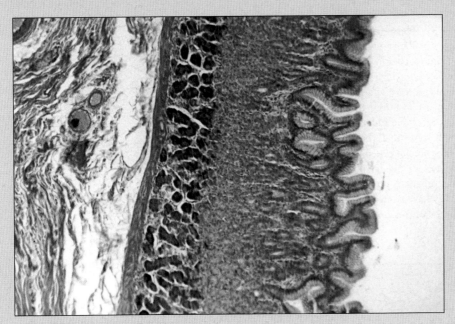

Figure 16-15 (50×): Fundic stomach.

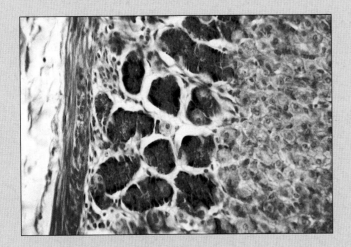

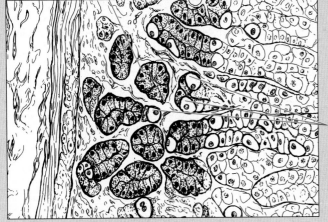

Parietal cell

Chief cells

Figure 16-16 (50×): Fundic stomach.

Pyloric Stomach

The pyloric stomach contains simple, branched, tubular pyloric glands, several of which open into each pit (**Figure 16-17**). The pyloric glands are more tortuous than those of the cardiac or fundic regions; therefore, in any given section, more of the tubules will be in transverse or oblique section. In addition, the majority of the cells within the pyloric glands resemble mucous neck cells. Closer examination, however, will show that these cells are taller than mucous neck cells, and their nuclei generally are orientated parallel to the longitudinal axis of the gland. Again, the transition from fundic to pyloric stomach is gradual. Therefore the pyloric section on your slide may have some characteristics that are intermediate between these two regions.

Small Intestine

General Histological Description of the Small Intestine

The small intestine is subdivided into three regions: duodenum, jejunum, and ileum. Histologically you can differentiate among these regions by comparing several distinct characteristics. The general characteristics of the small intestine are discussed first and should be studied using at least two of the photomicrographs in this section of the text. Only after these general characteristics are mastered should you proceed to the differences among the regions. In comparing the regions of the small intestine it is important for you to examine the photomicrographs in the order in which they are presented because the discussions build on each other.

Begin your examination of the small intestine with **Figure 16-18**. If you were to open the small intestine by a longitudinal incision you would see a series of definite folds running parallel to each other and passing in circular or oblique directions on the inner surface of the jejunum. These specializations of the mucosa are known as *plicae circulares*. The mucosa is further carried into a series of finger-like projections termed *villi*, which cover the entire surface of the plicae and small intestine. (Note: As you examine **Figure 16-18**, explain why some of the villi are represented in longitudinal section, whereas others are seen as cross section within the lumen of the organ.)

The *mucosa* also possesses numerous depressions termed *intestinal crypts* (or crypts of Lieberkuhn), which open between the villi and extend as deep as the muscularis mucosae. The simple, columnar epithelial cells of the mucosa possess a single basal nucleus and an apical brush border. Interspersed between the columnar epithelial cells you will find a varying number of goblet cells.

The *muscularis mucosa* is thin and composed of inner circular and outer longitudinal smooth muscle layers.

The *submucosa* is dense, irregular connective tissue (see section on Dense Irregular Connective Tissue in Chapter 3) containing nerves, blood vessels, and lymphoid nodules (see discussion of Diffuse Lymphoid Tissue and Lymphoid Nodules in Chapter 11).

The *muscularis externa* possesses two layers of smooth muscle: an inner, circularly arranged layer and an outer, longitudinally arranged layer.

As with the stomach, as you examine the histology of the small intestine you must direct your attention to two main questions:

- What histological characteristics will differentiate the small intestine from other hollow organs of the gastrointestinal tract?

- What histological characteristics will allow you to differentiate among the different regions of the small intestine?

Duodenum of the Small Intestine

In the duodenum you will note that the *villi* are rather low, broad, and leaf-like (**Figure 16-18**). Plicae circulares (not visible in this section) may or may not be seen in your section because the plicae are absent in the upper regions of the duodenum, as they begin to make their appearance near the junction with the jejunum.

There are several histological features that enable you to differentiate the duodenum from other regions of the small intestine (**Figure 16-18**):

- *Duodenal submucosal glands* (also called *Brunner's glands*): Duodenal glands will be found within the submucosa of the duodenum. These are highly branched, mucous-secreting, compound tubular glands lined by a simple columnar epithelium. The ducts pass up through the muscularis mucosae and lamina propria to empty into an intestinal crypt. Although most sections of the duodenum contain duodenal glands, you must keep in mind that the most inferior portions of the duodenum may contain a reduced number of these glands; therefore they may be absent from your section.

- *The number of goblet cells:* Goblet cells increase in number as you progress from the duodenum to the jejunum and ileum. Of the three regions of the small intestine, the duodenum therefore will have the fewest number of goblet cells and the ileum will have the most.

- *Shape of the villi:* As mentioned earlier, the villi of the duodenum are rather low, broad, and leaf-like. Although the difference in the shape of the villi is difficult to distinguish at first, this is a good histological feature that may be used to confirm your identification of the specimen.

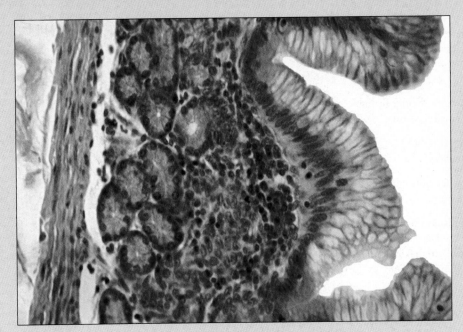

Figure 16-17 (100×): Pyloric stomach.

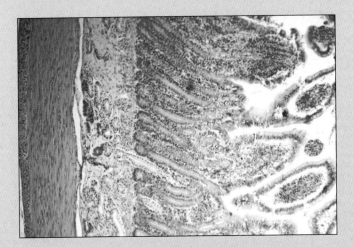

Figure 16-18 (25×): Duodenum of the small intestine.

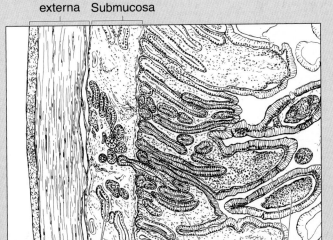

Muscularis
externa   Submucosa

Duodenal submucosal
gland

Intestinal
crypts

Villi

Jejunum of the Small Intestine

This photomicrograph shows the wall of the jejunum of the small intestine (**Figure 16-19**). Identification of the jejunum is based on the following characteristics:

- *Shape of the villi:* The villi are taller and more slender in the jejunum than in any other region of the small intestine.

- *Plicae circulares:* The jejunum demonstrates a more extensive development of the plicae circulares.

- *Number of goblet cells:* You note more goblet cells in the mucosa of the jejunum than in the duodenum.

- *Absence of duodenal glands:* The jejunum lacks duodenal glands and, as you have already learned, the absence of a structure may sometimes be just as valuable in making a correct identification as is the presence of another histological structure.

Ileum of the Small Intestine

Figure 16-20 shows the mucosa and submucosa of the ileum of the small intestine. Following are four major identifying features that help to differentiate the histology of the ileum from that of the duodenum and jejunum:

- *Shape of the villi:* Within the ileum you will find short, club-shaped villi.

- *Plica circulares:* The plicae are reduced in size in the ileum.

- *Number of goblet cells:* You will find a greater accumulation of goblet cells within the mucosal epithelium of the ileum than in any other region of the small intestine.

- *Aggregated Lymphoid Nodules:* You will note the presence of aggregated lymphoid nodules (also termed *Peyer's Patches*) (see section on Aggregated Lymphoid Nodules in Chapter 11) within the lamina propria. These patches are an aggregation of lymphoid nodules on the side of the ileum opposite the attachment of the mesentery.

On gross dissection of the ileum you will note that the mucosa immediately superficial to the aggregated lymphoid nodules is devoid of villi. Histological examination of that portion of the mucosa demonstrates that a single layer of columnar epithelium (without goblet cells) separates the nodules from the gut lumen. (Note: Is this visible in **Figure 16-20**? If not, what would be an accurate, histological reason for the appearance of this photomicrograph?)

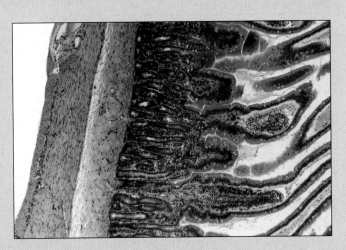

Figure 16-19 (25×): Jejunum of the small intestine.

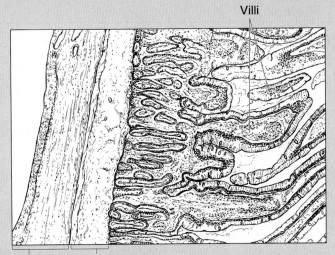

Villi

Muscularis Submucosa
externa

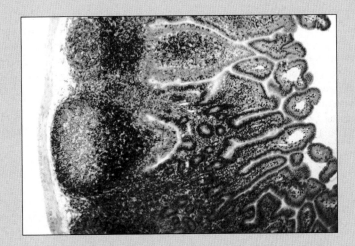

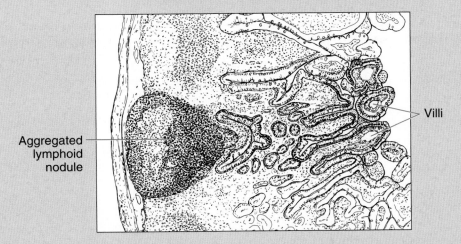

Aggregated
lymphoid
nodule

Villi

Figure 16-20 (25×): Ileum of the small intestine.

Colon

Figure 16-21 shows the mucosa and submucosa of the colon (large intestine). Note the fixation artifact that has caused a significant increase in the depth of the submucosa.

The *mucosa* of the large intestine is comparatively smooth when compared with that of the small intestine in that the large intestine lacks plicae or villi. The surface epithelium of the large intestine is composed of a simple columnar epithelium with numerous *goblet cells*.

Long, straight, tubular *glands* extend from the surface down through the entire thickness of the mucosa. The lamina propria of the mucosa is reduced to a minimum because of the close proximity of the glands. Solitary lymphoid nodules (see section on Lymphoid Nodules in Chapter 11) and isolated lymphocytes may be seen in the lamina propria of some preparations.

A *muscularis mucosae* composed of inner, circularly arranged and outer, longitudinally arranged smooth muscle is present. The *submucosa* is composed of dense, irregular connective tissue.

In humans, the muscularis externa (not visible on this photomicrograph) contains a complete inner, circular layer of smooth muscle and an outer, incomplete layer of longitudinally arranged smooth muscle termed the *taeniae coli*. Why is the arrangement of the muscularis externa not a reliable diagnostic feature for the colon?

The serosa (not visible in this photomicrograph) is a thin layer of connective tissue covered by a mesothelium.

As you compare the histology of the large intestine to that of the three regions of the small intestine, the following characteristics will serve as major identification features for the colon:

- *Number of goblet cells:* The mucosa of the large intestine has a significantly greater number of goblet cells than any region of the small intestine.

- *Lack of villi and plicae circulares:* The mucosa of the large intestine does not possess surface villa or plicae circulares.

- *Absence of duodenal glands and aggregated lymphoid nodules:* Although these structures are not found in every region of the small intestine, their absence in a specimen, when combined with the other characteristics mentioned above, may aid in confirming your identification of the large intestine.

Anorectal Junction

The histology of the rectum is nearly identical to that of the colon in that the same layers and sublayers are present. However, the rectum demonstrates at least four subtle differences when compared with the colon, as follows:

- The mucosa is deeper than that of the colon.

- The mucosal glands of the rectum are shorter than those of the colon.

- More goblet cells are present in mucosa of the rectum.

- The proximal (upper) portion of the rectum possesses transverse rectal folds.

The anal canal, which is distal to the rectum, may be subdivided into the following three regions or zones:

- Colorectal zone: This area possesses a mucosa composed of a simple columnar epithelium similar to that seen within the distal segments of the colon. The colorectal zone occupies approximately the proximal one third of the anal canal.

- Anal transitional zone: This zone occupies the middle one third of the anal canal and demonstrates a transitional region between the simple columnar epithelium of the colon and the stratified squamous epithelium of the perianal skin. The anal transitional zone possesses a stratified columnar epithelium.

- Squamous zone: Here the mucosal epithelium is a stratified squamous epithelium that becomes continuous with the skin of the perianal region.

Figure 16-22 demonstrates an area of transition between the rectal and anal canals.

The proximal (upper) portion of the anal canal also possesses longitudinal folds, termed *anal columns*, which are not visible on this photomicrograph. If anal columns are visible on your specimen, the depressions between the anal columns are termed *anal sinuses*.

If the muscularis externa is present on your specimen, you will note a marked thickening, which represents the internal anal sphincter (not visible on this photomicrograph).

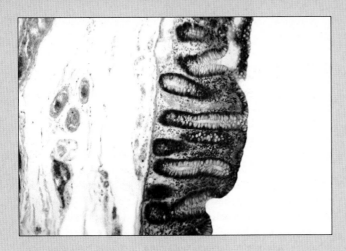

Figure 16-21 (25×): Colon.

Submucosa   Mucosa

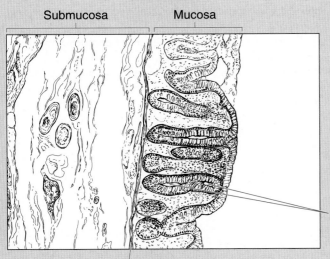

Intestinal
gland

Muscularis
mucosae

Anus   Rectum

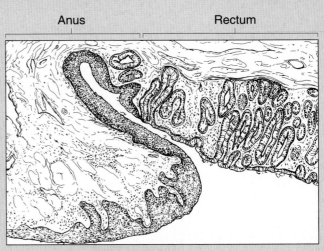

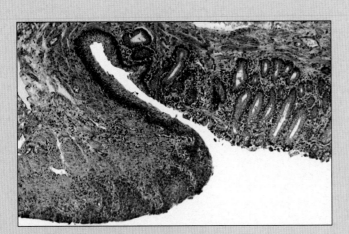

Figure 16-22 (25×): Rectal-anal junction.

Appendix

As you begin your examination of the appendix (Figure 16-23), the first thing you will notice is that *the lumen of the appendix varies in size and shape, and is frequently occluded as a result of fibrosis in adults.* However, if a patent lumen is present, it is small and cleft-like in cross section. The shape of the lumen may also change with age, being three-horned in youth and slit-like, circular, or another shape in the adult.

Further examination demonstrates that the appendix possesses the same four layers as the other tubular organs of the digestive tract (Figure 16-23). The *mucosa* of the appendix lacks villi and is composed of a simple columnar epithelium, crypts, a lamina propria, and a muscularis mucosae. The *glands* of the appendix may be more branched than those of the colon.

The lamina propria contains a large amount of lymphoid tissue in the form of numerous lymphoid nodules that, like the shape of the lumen, is a major histological feature of the appendix. In addition, the muscularis mucosae is poorly developed because of the large amount of lymphoid tissue.

Numerous adipose cells may be found within the *submucosa.*

The *muscularis externa* contains two complete layers of smooth muscle: an inner, circularly arranged layer and an outer, longitudinally arranged layer.

A typical serosa is present but may not be visible on your preparation.

Gallbladder

The wall of the gallbladder (Figure 16-24) is composed of only three layers; this is a major histological feature of this organ.

The *mucosa* has numerous folds that divide the surface into irregular polygonal areas. The surface epithelium is composed of simple columnar cells with oval nuclei. *Mucosal crypts* (also termed *Rokitansky-Aschoff sinuses*) *are another major histological feature of the gallbladder.* These are diverticula of the mucosa that extend into the muscular and perimuscular areas. The epithelium of these sinuses is a continuation of the surface epithelium.

The *lamina propria* is composed of loose, irregularly arranged (areolar) connective tissue containing extensive vascular plexuses and a few scattered muscle cells. *A muscularis mucosae and submucosa are lacking.*

The *muscularis externa* is composed of interlacing bundles of smooth muscle. Longitudinal fibers will be found closer to the lamina propria, whereas the remainder of the muscularis externa is circularly arranged. Connective tissue is found between the individual bundles.

A typical serosa is found external to the muscularis but only on the surface that is not attached to the liver.

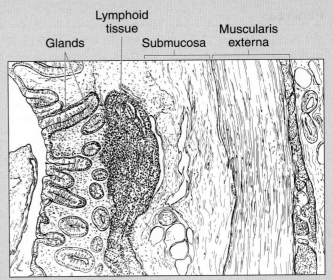

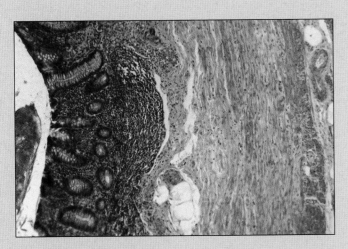

Figure 16-23 (25×): Appendix.

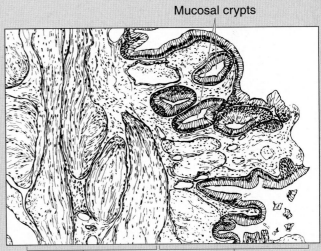

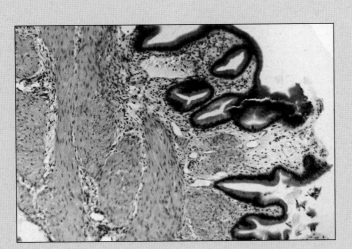

Figure 16-24 (25×): Gallbladder.

Pancreas

The pancreas (Figure 16-25) is a compound tubuloacinar gland with both endocrine and exocrine functions. The organ is covered with a thin layer of loose, irregularly arranged (areolar) connective tissue, not visible in this photomicrograph, and typically is not seen on histological preparations. No true capsule is present. Delicate *septa* radiate inward, subdividing the organ into lobules.

The duct system of the pancreas is composed of intercalated ducts, intralobular ducts, interlobular ducts, and the main pancreatic duct. The pancreas is unique in that the intercalated ducts, which are not visible on this photomicrograph, actually begin within the acini of the pancreas. Centroacinar cells (not visible on this photomicrograph), which are the initial cells of the intercalated ducts, are located within the serous acini of the pancreas. These ducts are quite short and drain into the intralobular ducts of the pancreas (not visible on this photomicrograph).

Intralobular ducts drain into *interlobular ducts*, which are lined with a tall, simple cuboidal or simple columnar epithelium resting on a distinct basal lamina (see section on Epithelial Sheets in Chapter 2). Occasionally goblet cells may also be found in the epithelium of these interlobular ducts.

The main excretory duct of the pancreas extends the entire length of the organ, receiving small branches, typically one per lobule. These lobular ducts (not visible in this photomicrograph) are lined by a simple cuboidal epithelium.

Pancreatic *acini* are all serous in composition. These acini possess a minute central lumen that may or may not be seen on high-dry objective, depending on the plane of section of your specimen.

At this time you should also review the histological discussion of the endocrine pancreas (see the section on the Endocrine Pancreas in Chapter 13), as well as **Figure 13-13.**

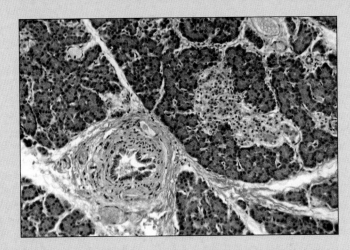

Figure 16-25 (25×): Pancreas.

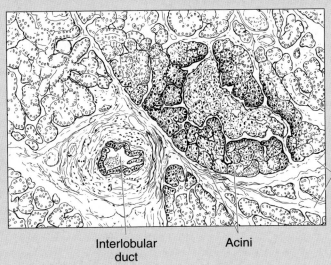

Septa

Interlobular
duct

Acini

Central vein

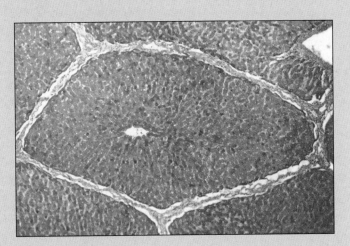

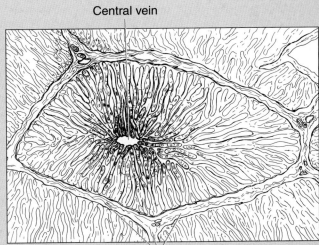

Figure 16-26 (25×): Liver.

Septa

Liver

The specimen in the following photomicrographs was obtained from a pig and is used to demonstrate more clearly the connective tissue of the hepatic lobule. Distinct connective tissue septa, dividing the liver into clearly defined lobules, is not seen in most animals, including humans.

Histologists may use any one of three ways to discuss the functional unit of the liver—the liver acinus, portal lobule, or classic lobule. The classic lobule is the one described in this text because it is traditionally used to describe the liver and is also the easiest to visualize with the light microscope. The structure of the classic lobule is based on the branches of the portal vein and hepatic artery, as well as the pathway that blood would follow as it perfuses the parenchyma of the liver.

The liver is contained within a delicate connective tissue capsule (not visible in this photomicrograph and typically not seen on histological preparations) from which delicate *septa* radiate inward, forming the framework for the parenchyma and dividing the liver into *lobules* (**Figure 16-26**). At the hilus, the capsule surrounds the entering and exiting blood vessels.

The classic hepatic lobule (see **Figure 16-26**) has a *central vein* from which liver parenchymal cells, termed *hepatocytes*, radiate outward like spokes of a wheel. *Hepatocytes* are arranged into irregular, branching, and interconnected plates termed *hepatic cords* (**Figure 16-27**). These hepatocytes are polyhedral in form, with sharply defined lateral and basal borders. The single central nucleus possesses one or more prominent nucleoli. Although they are not visible in this photomicrograph, when adjacent hepatocytes are viewed under oil immersion bile canaliculi may be visible as a small, pale, circular profile.

At the periphery of the classic liver lobule you will find *hepatic triads* (**Figure 16-27**) contained within the connective tissue of the lobule. The hepatic triad contains an *interlobular bile duct, interlobular artery* (which is a branch of the hepatic artery), and an *interlobular vein* (a tributary to the hepatic portal vein). A *lymphatic vessel* may also be present. The interlobular bile duct is easily recognized by its simple cuboidal epithelium. The interlobular artery and vein exhibit the characteristic histological characteristics of arteries and veins (see sections on Arteries and Veins in Chapter 8).

Hepatic sinusoids are abundant between the hepatocytes. These sinusoids make up the intralobular system of capillaries bathing the hepatic cords. By using either the high-dry or oil-immersion objective, you should be able to discern the thin endothelial layer making up the walls of the sinusoids. Between the hepatocytes and sinusoids is a connective tissue space of variable dimensions. This space is termed the *perisinusoidal space* (also termed the *space of Disse*), which is known to contain reticular fibers, occasional perisinusoidal cells, Kupffer cells (macrophages), and hepatocytic microvilli.

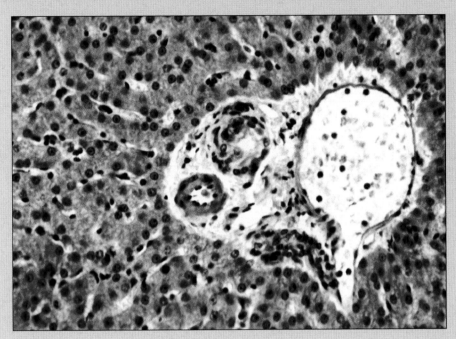

Figure 16-27 (100×): Hepatic triad within the liver.

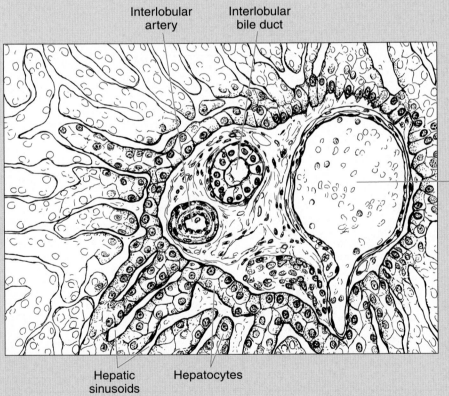

Interlobular artery

Interlobular bile duct

Interlobular vein

Hepatic sinusoids

Hepatocytes

Logic Tree

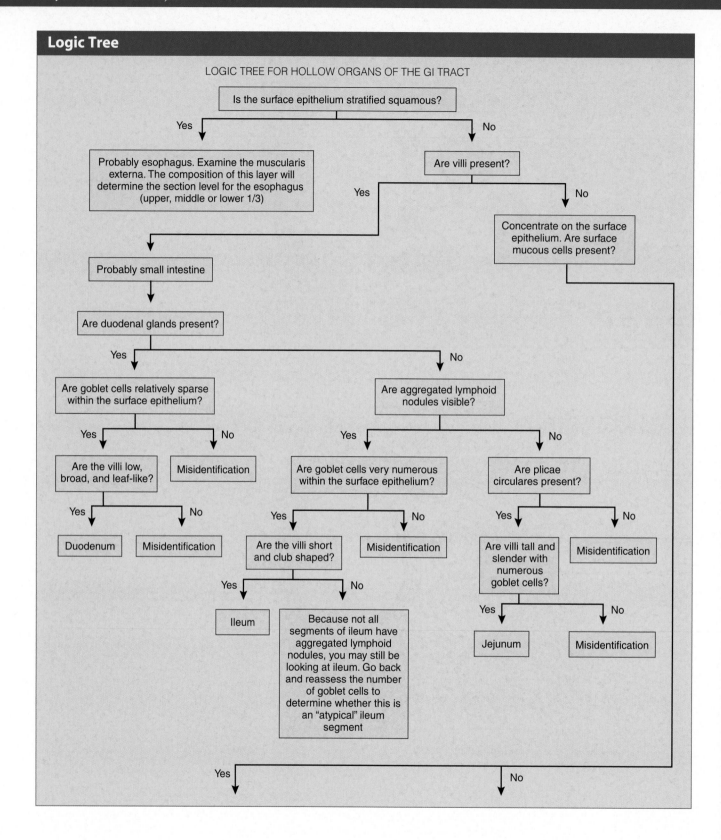

LOGIC TREE FOR HOLLOW ORGANS OF THE GI TRACT

Logic Tree

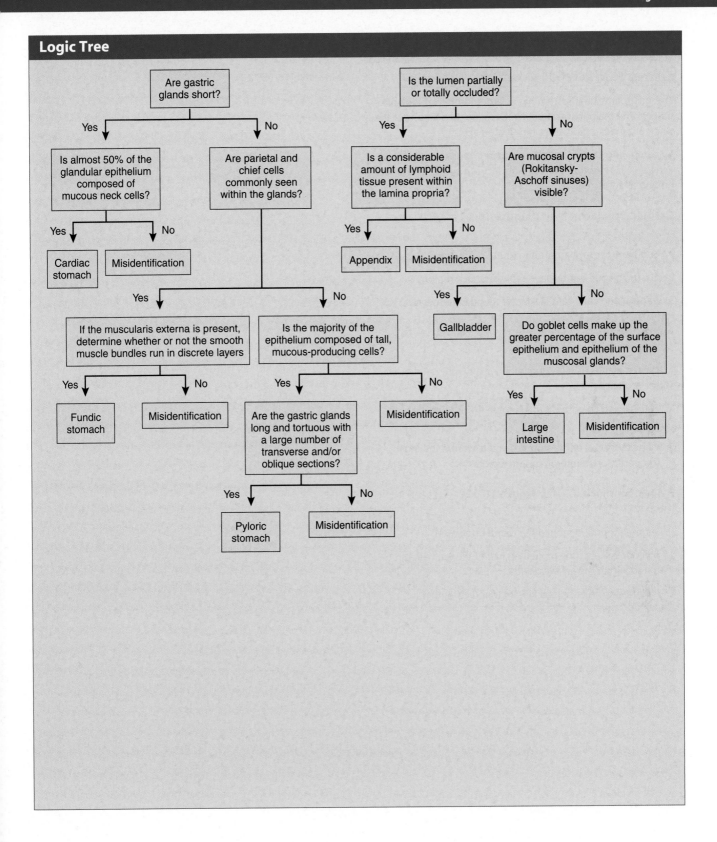

Commonly Misidentified Tissues

Cardiac, Fundic, and Pyloric Stomach

The gastrointestinal system has a large number of look-alike tissues. The majority of these involve different sections of the same organ (e.g., cardiac vs. fundic stomach).

By comparing cardiac, fundic, and pyloric regions of the stomach you will note that there are distinct but subtle differences among all three regions.

Cardiac Stomach (Review **Figure 16-14** in section on the Cardiac Stomach)

1. Segment of esophagus often found on section

2. Gastric glands shorter than other stomach regions

3. Parietal and chief cells lacking or found infrequently

Fundic Stomach (Review **Figures 16-15** and **16-16** in section on the Fundic Stomach)

1. Gastric glands usually longer than in any other region of the stomach

2. Parietal and chief cells prominent in lower portions of the gland

3. Largest portion of the stomach and therefore the most frequently encountered gastric region

Pyloric Stomach (Review **Figure 16-17** in section on the Pyloric Stomach)

1. Segment of duodenum often found on section

2. Mucous cells occupy more than half of the epithelium found within the gastric glands

3. Parietal and chief cells lacking or found infrequently

Commonly Misidentified Tissues

Duodenum, Jejunum, and Ileum of Small Intestine

As with the different regions of the stomach, the three regions of the small intestine possess distinct but subtle differences that enable histological differentiation. By comparing these sections, the following histological distinctions will become more apparent:

Duodenum (Review **Figure 16-18** in section on the Duodenum of the Small Intestine)

1. Duodenal glands present within submucosa
2. Fewest number of goblet cells
3. Villi appear leaf-like
4. Typically no lymphoid tissue within lamina propria

Jejunum (Review **Figure 16-19** in section on the Jejunum of the Small Intestine)

1. Duodenal glands absent
2. Goblet cells intermediate in number
3. Villi appear rounded
4. Typically no lymphoid tissue within lamina propria

Ileum (Review **Figure 16-20** in section on the Ileum of the Small Intestine)

1. Aggregated lymphoid nodules typically found within lamina propria
2. Highest number of goblet cells
3. Duodenal glands absent
4. Villi appear club shaped

Gallbladder and Small Intestine

The beginning (and often advanced) histology student may have difficulty differentiating between the gallbladder and small intestine. This difficulty usually results from the student's mistaking the convoluted folds of the mucosa of the gallbladder for intestinal villi. To prevent this error you should keep in mind the following characteristics of these two GI organs:

Gallbladder (Review **Figure 16-24** in section on the Gallbladder)

1. Mucosal folds resembling villi, but no true villi present
2. Lack of goblet cells
3. Muscularis thin and composed of interdigitating layers
4. Presence of mucosal crypts (Rokitansky-Aschoff sinuses)

Small Intestine (Review **Figures 16-18–16-20**)

1. True mucosal villi
2. Presence of goblet cells in surface epithelium
3. Muscularis externa quite thick and composed of two distinct layers (inner circular and outer longitudinal)
4. Lack of mucosal sinusoids

Commonly Misidentified Tissues

Lip and Vagina

As mentioned in Chapter 15, yet another problem may arise when trying to differentiate between lip and vaginal sections. Therefore you should review these differences between the two sections:

Lip (Review **Figure 16-1** in the section on the Lips)

1. Presence of hair follicles in dermis of facial skin

2. Possible presence of keratin in superficial layers of epidermis

3. Mucous glands present (labial glands)

4. Skeletal muscle present

5. Arteries dominant blood vessel

6. Collagen distinct within connective tissue

Vagina (Review **Figure 15-16** in the section on the Vagina in Chapter 15)

1. Absence of hair follicles

2. Smooth muscle present

3. Labial glands absent

4. Venous sinuses dominant blood vessel type

5. Collagen within connective tissue indistinct

Commonly Misidentified Tissues

Pancreas and Parotid Salivary Gland

Another common misidentification involves the pancreas and parotid salivary gland. Both of these glands have a serous acinar composition and at first glance are quite similar in histological appearance. Therefore you should try to keep the following differences in mind to aid in your identification:

Pancreas (Review **Figure 13-13** in section on the Endocrine Pancreas/Pancreatic Islets in Chapter 13 and **Figure 16-25** in section on the Pancreas)

1. Lightly staining pancreatic islets (Islets of Langerhans) present

2. Presence of centroacinar cells

3. Few adipose cells

Parotid Gland (Review **Figures 16-5** and **16-6** in section on the Parotid Salivary Gland)

1. Lack of pancreatic islets (Islets of Langerhans)

2. Lack of centroacinar cells

3. Numerous adipose cells

Chapter 17

INTEGUMENTARY SYSTEM

Chapter Objectives

This chapter will enable you to identify:

1. The various histological characteristics found in each layer of thin and thick skin

2. The various histological characteristics of pigmented skin

3. A lamellar corpuscle and a tactile corpuscle

Before you begin to study the histological characteristics of the skin and its derivatives, it is important for you to review the anatomy of the various layers of the skin, as well as the functions of these layers.

Thick Skin

Thick skin (Figure 17-1), which lacks hair, is found on the palms of the hands and the soles of the feet. The most superficial layer of the *epidermis* is termed the *stratum corneum*. This is a rather thick layer composed of clear, dead, scale-like cells termed *keratinocytes*. They have a thickened cellular membrane and no nuclei, and they are closely interdigitated. The cytoplasm has been replaced by keratin proteins.

Deep to the stratum corneum is the *stratum lucidum*, a rather thin layer that has staining characteristics different from those of the stratum corneum. (In this photomicrograph, the stratum lucidum stains significantly darker than the more superficial stratum corneum.)

The *stratum granulosum* is found deep to the stratum lucidum and is composed of two to five rows of flattened, lightly staining cells, the longitudinal axes of which run parallel to the surface. Cells of this layer contain numerous cytoplasmic granules that usually stain intensely with hematoxylin.

The cells of the next two layers possess quite similar histological characteristics. Their nuclei are deeply chromatic, whereas the cytoplasm is deeply basophilic and contains numerous fine filaments that are not visible with the light microscope. The cells of the *stratum spinosum*, which are found in the layer immediately deep to the stratum granulosum, are polygonal in shape and are held together closely by desmosomes. During fixation, the cells of this layer often pull apart, thereby creating the "spines," characteristic of this layer, that actually are fixation artifacts.

The deepest layer of the epidermis is the *stratum basale*. It is composed of a single layer of columnar or high cuboidal cells on a basal lamina (see description of basal lamina in section on Epithelial Sheets in Chapter 2). The shape of these cells varies from ovoid in the deepest layer to round in the cells closest to the stratum spinosum. These cells are somewhat smaller in overall size than those of the stratum spinosum.

The *dermis* of the skin is composed mostly of dense, irregular connective tissue (see section on Dense Irregular Connective Tissue [Dermis of the Skin] in Chapter 3) containing all three connective tissue fiber types. The dermis is subdivided into two layers: a deep *reticular layer* and a superficial *papillary layer*. The reticular layer is characterized by dense, collagenous fibers arranged into bundles that are often seen to unite to form secondary bundles that interlace frequently.

The papillary layer is composed of loose connective tissue (see section on Loose, Irregular Connective Tissue [Lamina Propria of Duodenum] in Chapter 3) with fine and closely arranged connective tissue fibers. *Papillae* are seen to indent the deepest layers of the epidermis. These papillae contain blood vessels (see section on Blood Vessels in Chapter 8) that nourish (but do not enter) the more superficial epidermal layers and peripheral nerves (see section on Peripheral Nerves in Chapter 7) that either terminate in the dermis or penetrate the basal lamina and enter the epidermis.

Thin Skin (Pigmented)

The terms *thick* and *thin* skin refer to the thickness of the epidermis. Thin skin lacks a stratum lucidum and therefore is composed of only four layers.

Thin skin (Figure 17-2) covers most of the body and usually possesses hair. However, thin skin that lacks hair may be found in the lips, terminal and lateral portions of the fingers and toes, and portions of the external genitalia. In thin skin, all of the layers are reduced in thickness, with the stratum corneum, stratum spinosum, and stratum basale being the only layers that are consistently represented in all parts of the body.

The color of the epidermis is due to a combination of the dermal blood supply, the thickness of the epidermis, and variable quantities of two pigments: *carotene* and *melanin*. Note the presence of *pigment granules* within the *keratinocytes* located in the deeper layers of the epidermis.

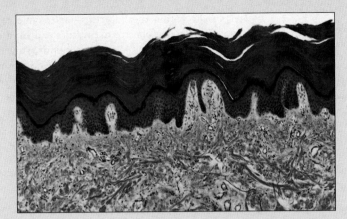

Figure 17-1 (25×): Thick skin (Caucasian).

Papilla   Papillary layer

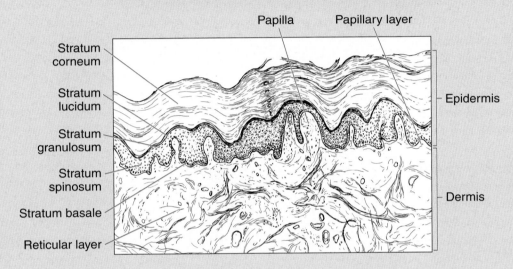

Stratum corneum

Stratum lucidum

Stratum granulosum

Stratum spinosum

Stratum basale

Reticular layer

Epidermis

Dermis

Figure 17-2 (25×): Thin skin (pigmented).

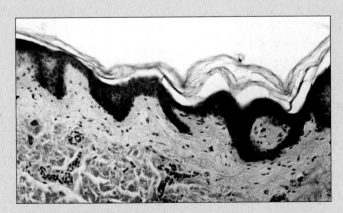

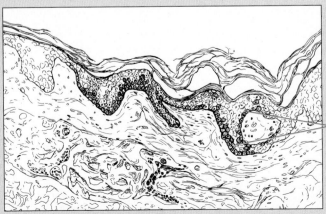

Keratinocytes

Scalp

Hairy scalp contains *hair follicles* and their associated *sebaceous glands* and *arrector pili muscle* (Figure 17-3).

Lamellar and Tactile Corpuscles

Lamellar Corpuscle

Lamellar (also termed *pacinian*) *corpuscles* (Figure 17-4) are found in association with joints, internal organs, periosteum of bones, the hypodermis, and the deeper layers of the skin—especially within the fingertips—and connective tissue in general. They are responsive to pressure and vibratory stimuli.

A lamellar corpuscle is composed of a myelinated axon surrounded by a capsular structure. As the neuron enters the corpuscle, its myelin covering remains intact for only one to three nodal segments. Then the myelin is replaced by flattened Schwann cells that will form the inner core of the capsule. Around this inner core are concentric lamellae composed of flattened cells similar to those found within the endoneurium of peripheral nerves. Delicate collagenous fibers, a few isolated capillaries, and fluid fill the space between these lamellae.

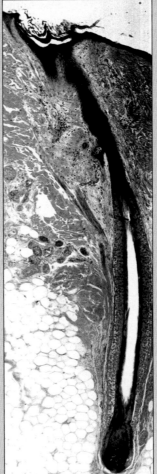

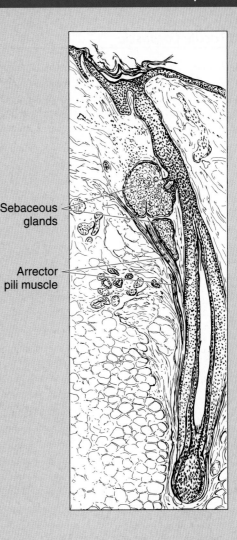

Figure 17-3 (25×): Scalp demonstrating a hair follicle.

Sebaceous glands

Arrector pili muscle

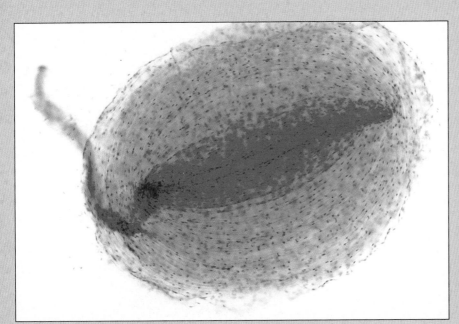

Figure 17-4 (70×): Lamellar corpuscle.

Tactile Corpuscle

Tactile corpuscles (also termed *Meissner's corpuscles*) (Figures 17-5 and 17-6) are touch receptors found within hairless skin. They are especially numerous in the lips, hands (palmar surface and fingers), soles of the feet, and the undersurface of the toes. These structures are typically found just deep to the stratum basale within the dermal papillae and are orientated perpendicular to the surface of the skin.

Tactile corpuscles resemble a tapered cylinder. They are composed of one or two sensory nerves that penetrate the corpuscle and spiral within a cellular component of flattened Schwann cells, which then form several irregular lamellae around the sensory nerves.

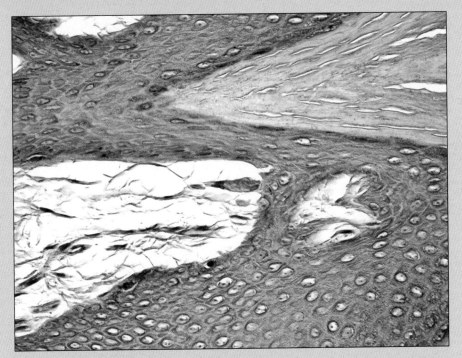

Figure 17-5 (70×): Tactile corpuscle.

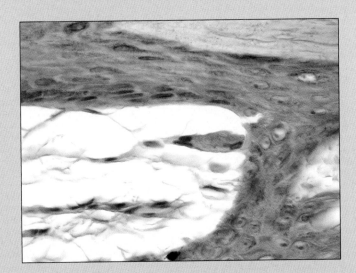

Figure 17-6 (140×): Tactile corpuscle.

Peripheral nerve   Tactile corpuscle

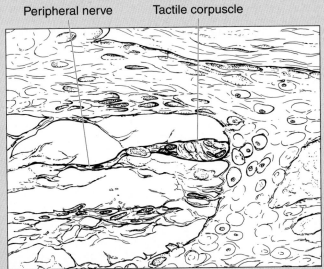

Chapter 18

SPECIAL SENSES

Chapter Objectives

This chapter will enable you to identify the histological characteristics of the:

1. Olfactory epithelium of the nose
2. Cornea of the eye
3. Retina of the eye
4. Cochlea of the ear

Olfactory Epithelium

The cells responsible for the sense of smell are located within the posterodorsal regions of the nasal cavities. The olfactory epithelium is pigmented yellowish-brown, in contrast to the pinkish color of the respiratory epithelium. This yellowish-brown color is due to the presence of glands within the olfactory epithelium and pigment within the olfactory epithelial cells.

Olfactory epithelium (Figures 18-1 and 18-2) is similar to that of the respiratory tree (see section on Pseudostratified Epithelia in Chapter 2) in that it is a pseudostratifed columnar epithelium. However, the olfactory epithelium is lacking goblet cells and ciliated epithelial cells. The olfactory epithelium is composed of four cell types:

- Olfactory cells, which are bipolar neurons that span the entire thickness of the epithelium

- Supporting (sustentacular cells)

- Basal cells (stem cells)

- Brush cells, which are similar to those found within the respiratory epithelium

Deep to the olfactory epithelium you will see numerous capillaries, *olfactory glands*, unmyelinated and myelinated neurons. The lamina propria of the olfactory epithelium is continuous with the perichondrium or periosteum of the nasal cavity.

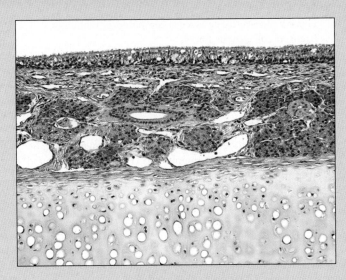

Figure 18-1 (35×): Olfactory epithelium.

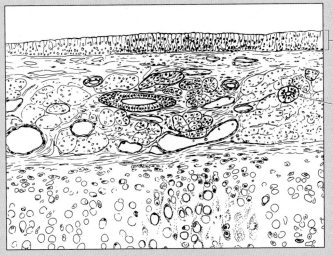

Olfactory epithelium

Olfactory gland

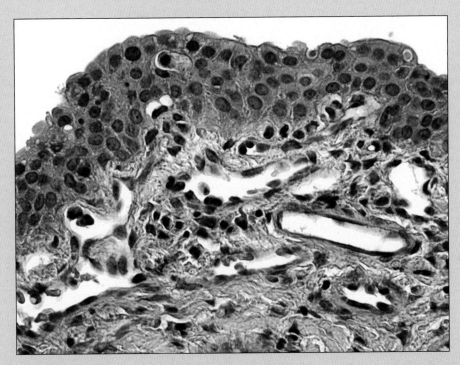

Figure 18-2 (70×): Olfactory epithelium.

Eye

Cornea

The cornea of the eye is a part of the fibrous tunic and is continuous with the sclera. Because the cornea is avascular, the superficial structures must obtain oxygen and nutrients from the tears that bathe its anterior surface.

The cornea is composed of five layers:

- *The corneal epithelium* (anterior epithelium) (Figures 18-3 and 18-4) is a stratified, nonkeratinized squamous epithelium.

- An *anterior limiting membrane* (Bowman's membrane) (Figures 18-3 and 18-4) lies deep to the corneal epithelium.

This connective tissue layer is composed of randomly arranged collagenous fibers.

- The *substantia propria* (corneal stroma) (Figures 18-3 and 18-4) is a thick layer of parallel bundles of collagen fibers interspersed with fibrocytes. Each layer of connective tissue bundles within the substantial propria lies perpendicular to its adjacent layer.

- A *posterior limiting membrane* (Descemet's membrane, or the posterior basement membrane) (Figure 18-3) is found deep to the substantia propria. This layer serves as the basal lamina for the *endothelium of the anterior chamber.*

- The *endothelium of the anterior chamber* (posterior epithelium) (Figure 18-3) is a simple squamous epithelium that faces the anterior chamber of the eye.

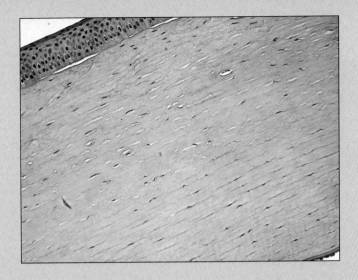

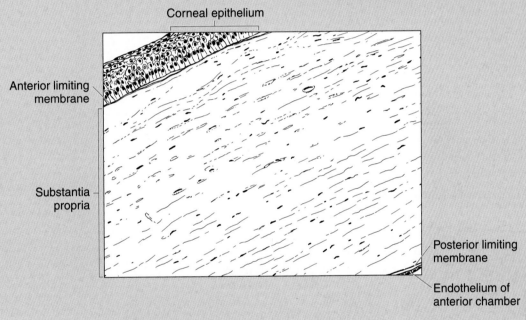

Figure 18-3 (35×): Cornea.

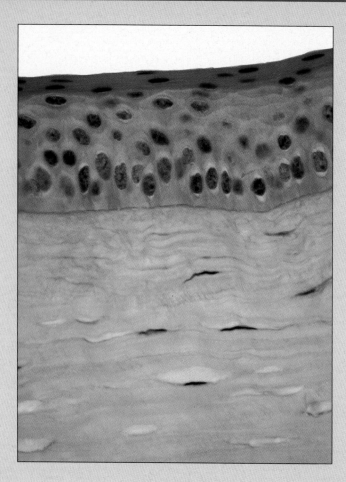

Figure 18-4 (40×): Cornea.

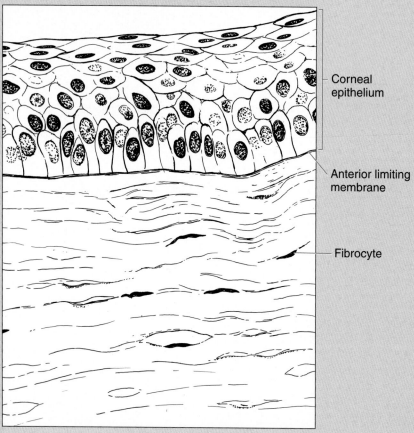

Corneal
epithelium

Anterior limiting
membrane

Fibrocyte

Retina

The retina of the eye consists of two layers: the neural retina (retina proper), which contains the photoreceptors, and the retinal pigment epithelium, an outer layer that is attached to the choroid.

The neural retina is also subdivided into two parts:

- The nonvisual retina, which is found anterior to the ora serrata

- The optic part of the retina, which contains the photoreceptors and lines the posterior surface of the eye

The optic portion of the retina is subdivided into 10 layers (Figures 18-5 and 18-6):

- The *pigment epithelium*, which rests on the lamina vitrea, is immediately superficial to the *choroid* and contains melanin-containing cells.

- Rods and cones

- Outer limiting membrane (not visible on this photomicrograph), which is a sieve-like sheet of connective tissue

- *Outer nuclear layer*, which contains the cell bodies of the rods and cones

- The outer plexiform layer (not visible on this photomicrograph), which contains the axonal processes of the rods and cones

- *The inner nuclear layer*, which contains the cell bodies of the bipolar cells (the first order neurons of the optic tract), supporting (Muller's) cells, horizontal cells, and amacrine cells

- The *inner plexiform layer*, which contains the neural processes of bipolar, supporting, horizontal, and amacrine cells

- The *ganglion cell* layer, which contains the soma of the ganglion cells, the second order neurons of the optic tract

- The *optic nerve layer*, which contains the neuronal processes of the ganglion cells that will ultimately form the optic nerve

- *Inner limiting membrane* layer, which is formed by the basal lamina of the Muller's cells

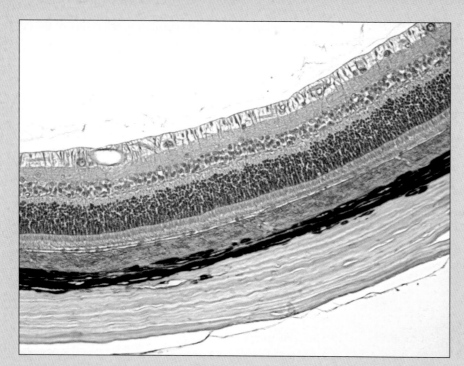

Figure 18-5 (35×): Retina.

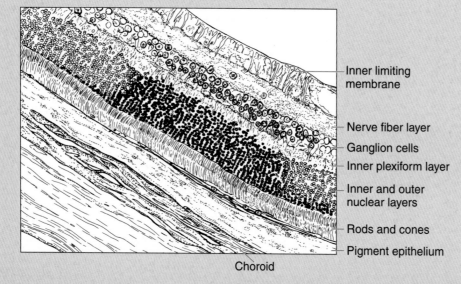

Figure 18-6 (70×): Retina.

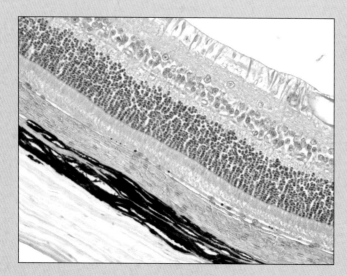

Inner limiting membrane

Nerve fiber layer

Ganglion cells

Inner plexiform layer

Inner and outer nuclear layers

Rods and cones

Pigment epithelium

Choroid

Organ of Corti of the Ear (Guinea Pig)

The Organ of Corti is the sensory structure of the auditory portion of the ear. It is found within the cochlear duct (scala media), which is within the membranous labyrinth of the inner ear. The membranous labyrinth is divided into three segments, or ducts (that are not labeled on this photomicrograph), by two membranes of the inner ear. The *basilar membrane* separates the cochlear duct (scala media) above from the tympanic duct (scala tympani) below. The *vestibular membrane* separates the cochlear duct below from the vestibular duct (scala vestibuli) above.

The Organ of Corti (Figure 18-7) rests on the *basilar membrane*, which separates the cochlear duct above from the tympanic duct below. *Hair cells* rest on the basilar membrane and are in contact with the *tectorial membrane*. (Note that the tectorial membrane is not intact in this photomicrograph, because of a sectioning artifact.)

Also visible on Figure 18-7 are the *spiral limbus* and the *stria vascularis* of the inner ear. The stria vascularis forms the outer wall of the cochlear duct and is a highly vascular area. A unique stratified epithelium that contains an intraepithelial capillary network covers the stria vascularis. The floor of the cochlear duct is partly formed by the spiral limbus, which is a thickened form of periosteal tissue.

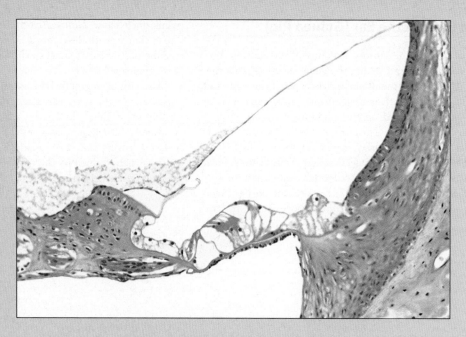

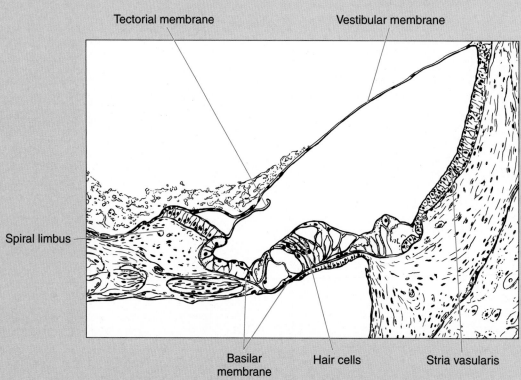

Tectorial membrane   Vestibular membrane

Spiral limbus

Basilar membrane   Hair cells   Stria vasularis

Figure 18-7 (70×): Organ of Corti.

NOTES ON HISTOLOGICAL TISSUE PREPARATIONS AND STAINING TECHNIQUES

Histology students must have some understanding of how histological specimens are prepared. This rudimentary understanding of tissue fixation and staining will enable students to understand the appearance of the finished product they will be studying.

Histological Tissue Preparation

The preparation of tissue for histological examination involves several steps:

1. Fixation: Tissue specimens are preserved in a variety of fixatives. The type of fixative chosen is determined by the type of tissue or organ to be studied and the various components found within that tissue or organ.

2. Embedding: After the tissue has been fixed it is firmly embedded into a medium that allows sectioning of the specimen at the desired thickness. Routine histological preparations are sectioned at a thickness of between 4 and 10 μm.

3. Staining: An unstained specimen typically does not possess sufficient contrast to enable someone to adequately distinguish organ, tissue, and cellular characteristics. Therefore tissues will be stained with some form of organic and inorganic compounds (histological stains) that will enable adequate differentiation of tissue components and cellular detail.

Histological Stains

Although most of the photomicrographs contained within this text are of specimens stained with hematoxylin and eosin (H & E), students of histology may encounter a wide variety of stains. The most commonly encountered stains and their characteristics are listed below.

Azan

Although typically considered a connective tissue stain, this stain may also be used to demonstrate the fine cytological detail of epithelial tissue. Nuclei of epithelial tissue will stain bright red, whereas collagen of the basal lamina will stain blue. If Azan is used with other tissues, mucin will stain blue; muscle and red blood cells will stain orange.

Hematoxylin & Eosin (H & E)

This is the most commonly encountered histological stain. Hematoxylin, a base, stains acidic cellular structures, including nuclei, ribosomes, and rough endoplasmic reticulum (RER) a blue to purplish-blue color. Eosin, an acid, stains predominantly basic structures pink or red. Such structures include membranous structures within a cell. Typically a cell that is actively synthesizing proteins will stain deeply basophilic, whereas a "resting" protein-synthesizing cell will stain eosinophilic. In addition, a cell with a large number of membranous components (such as the proximal convoluted tubule cells of the kidney) will stain eosinophilic.

Masson's Trichrome

This stain is typically used with connective tissue and produces three staining reactions: cytoplasm, muscle, erythrocytes, and keratin are stained red; basophilic structures (i.e., nuclei) are stained blue; and collagen is stained green.

Nissl and Methylene Blue Stains

A basic dye commonly used to demonstrate RER within neuronal somas.

Periodic Acid-Schiff Reaction (PAS)

Periodic Acid-Schiff Reaction (PAS) staining is a form of histochemical staining. Histochemical staining is used specifically to stain certain components of cells or tissues. PAS specifically stains complex carbohydrates a deep red color. PAS-positive components include cartilage, mucin of goblet cells, the basal lamina of renal tubules, and the brush borders of renal tubular cells.

Reticulin Stain

This stain most clearly demonstrates reticular fibers. When this stain is used, reticular fibers will stain black or dark blue.

Silver or Gold Impregnation

These "heavy metal" stains are typically used with nervous tissue to demonstrate cellular processes (axons and dendrites). Cells and cellular processes will appear back, brown, or golden when stained with either of these heavy metals.

Sudan Black and Osmium Stains

These brownish-black stains are is used to demonstrate lipid-containing structures, such as the myelin covering of neurons.

Wright Stain

This stain is commonly used for bone marrow and blood smears. With this stain, nuclei will be purple and cytoplasm will be a light blue. Depending on their composition, cytoplasmic granules will stain variably (usually purple, pink, or unstained).

Index

Page numbers followed by *f* indicate figures; *t*, tables

Urethra
  female, 174, 175f
  logic tree for, 177
  male, 170, 171f, 173f, 174, 177f
  prostatic, 170, 171f, 174, 177f, 205f
  spongy, 26, 27f, 170, 172, 173f, 174
Urethral glands, 170, 172, 174, 175f, 177f
Urinary bladder, 31f, 163, 168–171, 169f, 171f, 174, 177f
Urinary pole, 163, 165f
Urinary system
  bladder. *See* Urinary bladder
  functions of, 163
  kidneys. *See* Kidneys
  penis, 172, 173f
  ureter, 163, 168, 169f, 174, 177f, 226
  urethra. *See* Urethra
Uterine tubes, 218, 219f, 226
Uterus
  layers of, 218, 219f
  during menstrual cycle, 218–222, 221f, 223f

V

Vagina, 224, 225f, 264
Vallate papillae, 228, 230, 231f
Vasa recta, 168, 169f
Veins
  characteristics of, 118, 119f, 122, 123f
  trabecular, 158, 159f

Venous sinuses, 158, 161f
Venules, 121f, 122, 123f
Vestibular membrane, 281, 282f
Villi, 14, 15f, 17f, 145, 252
Volkmann's canal, 70

W

White adipose tissue, 46, 47f
White fat, 48
White matter, 89–90
White pulp, 158, 159f, 162f
Working distance of the lens, 2
Wright stain
  of basophilic granulocytes, 131f
  of eosinophilic granulocytes, 127t, 130, 131f
  of lymphocytes, 129f
  of monocytes, 129f
  of neutrophilic granulocytes, 133f
  of platelets, 126f
  of red blood cells, 126f

Z

Zona fasciculata, 188, 189f
Zona glomerulosa, 188, 189f
Zona pellucida, 212, 213f, 214, 215f
Zona reticularis, 188, 189f